Keep up-to-date a ☑ SO-BBH-609

Gain free access to new drug monographs, the latest FDA approvals, innovative articles on pharmacology, drug alerts, dangerous side effects, and potentially life threatening drug-drug, drug-natural product, and drug-food interactions.

Contents

drugguide.com

comprehensive drug
information on the web

Features of this site include:

- 5,000+ trade and generic drugs

- Over 1,700 drug monographs

- Customizable bookmarking

- Related topic cross-linking

- "Sounds like" searching

- Regular updates

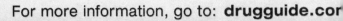

For more information, go to: **drugguide.com**

alvimopan (al-vi-mo-pan)
Entereg
Classification
Thera: gastric stimulants
Pharm: opioid antagonists

Pregnancy Category B

Indications

Speed time to upper/lower GI recovery following partial large/small bowel resection with primary anastamosis.

Action

Acts peripherally as μ-opioid receptor antagonist which speeds recovery of bowel function after to partial large or small bowel resection surgery with anastomosis surgery. **Therapeutic Effects:** Accelerated time to bowel recovery following primary anastamotic surgery.

Pharmacokinetics

Absorption: 6% absorbed following oral administration.
Distribution: Does not cross the blood-brain barrier.
Protein Binding: *alvimopan*—80% bound to albumin; *metabolite*—94% bound to albumin.
Metabolism and Excretion: Converted by bacterial flora in the GI tract to an active metabolite; elimination is mostly via biliary secretion, followed by conversion by bacterial flora. Elimination of unabsorbed drug and metabolites is via feces and urine.
Half-life: *alvimopan*—10–17 hr; *metabolite*—10–18 hr.

TIME/ACTION PROFILE (blood levels)

ROUTE	ONSET	PEAK	DURATION
PO	unknown	2 hr	12 hr

Contraindications/Precautions

Contraindicated in: Therapeutic doses of opioid analgesics for more than 7 consecutive days before initiation of alvimopan; Severe hepatic impairment or end-stage renal disease.
Use Cautiously in: More than 3 doses of opioids within the wk prior to surgery (↑ sensitivity to effects and adverse reactions including abdominal pain, nausea, vomiting and diarrhea); Mild to moderate hepatic or renal impairment (↑ risk of adverse effects); **Geri:** May have ↑ sensitivity to effects; **OB: Lactation:** Use in pregnancy only if clearly needed); use cautiously during lactation; **Pedi:** Safe use in children not established).

Adverse Reactions/Side Effects

GI: <u>constipation</u>, <u>dyspepsia</u>, <u>flatulence</u>. **F and E:** hypokalemia. **GU:** urinary retention. **Hemat:** anemia. **MS:** back pain.

Interactions

Drug-Drug: Previous (within 1 wk) **opioid** use ↑ risk of adverse reactions (avoid if therapeutic opioid doses used during prior wk, use cautiously if more than 3 doses have been used).

Route/Dosage

PO (Adults): 12 mg for 30 min–5 hr prior to surgery, then 12 mg twice daily for up to 15 doses.

Availability

Capsules: 12 mg.

NURSING IMPLICATIONS

Assessment

- Assess bowel sounds and frequency, quantity, and consistency of stools periodically during therapy.
- *Lab Test Considerations:* May cause anemia and hypokalemia.

Potential Nursing Diagnoses

Constipation (Indications)

Implementation

- Must be administered **only** during hospitalization. Only available in hospitals enrolled in the Entereg Access Support and Education (E.A.S.E.) program.
- **PO:** Administer twice daily without regard to food for no more than 7 days.

Patient/Family Teaching

- Explain purpose of alvimopan to patient.
- Advise patient to notify health care professional if they have taken long term or intermittent opioid pain therapy, including any use of opioids in the wk prior to receiving alvimopan.

Evaluation/Desired Outcomes

- Resolution of postoperative ileus following bowel resection.

---

bendamustine
(ben-da-**muss**-teen)
Treanda
Classification
Thera: antineoplastics
Pharm: benzimidazoles

Pregnancy Category D

Indications

Chronic lymphocytic leukemia. Indolent B-cell non-Hodgkin's lymphoma that has progressed during or within 6 mo of receiving rituximab or a rituximab-containing regimen.

Action

Damages DNA resulting in death of rapidly replicating cells. **Therapeutic Effects:** Decreased proliferation of leukemic cells. Death of lymphoma cells.

Pharmacokinetics

Absorption: IV administration results in complete bioavailability.

Distribution: Distributes freely into red blood cells.
Protein Binding: 94–96%.
Metabolism and Excretion: Mostly metabolized (partially by the CYP1A2 enzyme system; 90% excreted in feces; some renal elimination. Although metabolites have antineoplastic activity, levels are extremely low.
Half-life: 40 min.

TIME/ACTION PROFILE (blood levels)

ROUTE	ONSET	PEAK	DURATION
IV	rapid	end of infusion	unknown

Contraindications/Precautions

Contraindicated in: Hypersensitivity to bendamustine or mannitol; CCr <40 ml/min. Use with caution in lesser degrees of renal impairment; Moderate or severe hepatic impairment; **OB:** Pregnancy or lactation.
Use Cautiously in: Patients at risk for tumor lysis syndrome (concurrent allopurinol recommended); Mild hepatic impairment; Mild to moderate renal impairment; Patients with child-bearing potential; **Geri:** Elderly patients may be more susceptible to adverse reactions; **Pedi:** Safety not established.

Adverse Reactions/Side Effects

CNS: fatigue, weakness. **Resp:** cough. **GI:** nausea, vomiting, diarrhea. **Derm:** skin reactions. **Hemat:** anemia, LEUKOPENIA, NEUTROPENIA, THROMBOCYTOPENIA. **Metab:** hyperuricemia. **Misc:** MALIGNANCY, TUMOR LYSIS SYNDROME, allergic reactions including ANAPHYLAXIS, fever, infusion reactions.

Interactions

Drug-Drug: Concurrent use of **CYP1A2 inducers/inhibitors** can alter levels of bendamustine. **Inhibitors of CYP1A2** including **fluvoxamine** and **ciprofloxacin** may ↑ levels of bendamustine and ↓ levels of active metabolites. **Inducers of CYP1A2** including **omeprazole** and **smoking** may ↓ levels of bendamustine and ↑ levels of its active metabolites. Consider alternative treatments.

Route/Dosage

Chronic Lymphocytic Leukemia

IV (Adults): 100 mg/m² on days 1 and 2 of a 28 day cycle, up to 6 cycles; dose modification required for toxicity.

Non-Hodgkin's Lymphoma

IV (Adults): 120 mg/m² on days 1 and 2 of a 21 day cycle, up to 8 cycles; dose modification required for toxicity.

Availability

Lyophilized powder for injection (requires reconstitution): 100 mg vial.

NURSING IMPLICATIONS

Assessment

- Monitor for bone marrow depression. Assess for bleeding (bleeding gums, bruising, petechiae, guaiac stools, urine, and emesis) and avoid IM injections and taking rectal temperatures if platelet count is low. Apply pressure to venipuncture sites for 10 min. Assess for signs of infection during neutropenia. Anemia may occur; monitor for increased fatigue, dyspnea, and orthostatic hypotension.
- Monitor for symptoms of infusion reactions (fever, chills, pruritus, rash). May rarely cause severe allergic and anaphylactic reactions, especially in second and subsequent cycles. Discontinue therapy if severe reactions occur. Ask patient about symptoms suggestive of infusion reactions after first cycle of therapy. Consider using antihistamines, antipyretics, and corticosteroids in patients who previously experienced Grade 1 or 2 reactions. Consider discontinuation of therapy in patients with Grade 3 or 4 reactions.
- Assess for tumor lysis syndrome. Usually occurs during first cycle of bendamustine. May lead to acute renal failure and death. Maintain adequate volume status, close monitoring of blood chemistry, especially potassium and uric acid levels, and use allopurinol during first 1–2 wks of therapy in high risk patients.
- Assess for skin reactions (rash, toxic skin reactions, bullous exanthema). Withhold or discontinue therapy if reactions are progressive or severe If non-hematologic toxicity is ≥Grade 3, reduce dose to 50 mg/m² on Days 1 and 2 of each cycle.
- Monitor intake and output, appetite, and nutritional intake. Assess for nausea and vomiting. Administration of an antiemetic before and during therapy and adjusting diet as tolerated may help maintain fluid and electrolyte balance and nutritional status.
- *Lab Test Considerations:* Monitor CBC with differential and platelet count before and during therapy. The hematologic nadirs occur wk 3. Recovery usually occurs in 28 days. Withhold dose and notify physician if ANC in ≥1 × 10⁹/L and the platelet count is ≥ 75,000 × 10⁹/L. If hemotologic toxicity ≥ Grade 3, reduce dose to 50 mg/m² on Days 1 and 2. If Grade 3 or great toxicity recurs, reduce dose to 25 mg/m² on Days 1 and 2.
- Monitor blood chemistry, especially serum potassium and uric acid before and periodically during therapy. Allopurinol may be used during first wks of therapy to prevent tumor lysis syndrome.

Potential Nursing Diagnoses

Risk for infection (Side Effects)

Implementation

- **High Alert:** Fatalities have occurred with chemotherapeutic agents. Before administering, clarify all ambiguous orders; double check single, daily, and course-of-therapy dose limits; have second practitioner independently double check original order, calculations and infusion pump settings.

IV Administration

- Solution should be prepared in a biologic cabinet. Wear gloves and safety glasses while handling medication. Discard equipment in designated containers.
- **Intermittent Infusion:** Reconstitute each 100-mg vial with 20 ml of Sterile Water for Injection. Solution should be clear, colorless to pale yellow. Do not administer solutions that are discolored or contain a precipitate. **Concentration:** 5 mg/mL. **Diluent:** Withdraw volume needed and transfer to a 500 mL of 0.9% NaCl within 30 min of reconstitution. Mix thoroughly.
- Diluted solution is stable for 24 hr when refrigerated or 3 hr at room temperature; administration must be completed within this period. Solution contains no preservatives; discard unused solution. **Rate:** Administer over 30 min.
- **Additive Incompatibility:** Do not admix or dilute with other solutions or medication.

Patient/Family Teaching

- Instruct patient to notify health care professional if fever; chills; sore throat; signs of infection; lower back or side pain; difficult or painful urination; shortness of breath; fatigue; bleeding gums; bruising; petechiae; or blood in urine, stool, or emesis occurs. Caution patient to avoid crowds and persons with known infections. Instruct patient to use soft toothbrush and electric razor. Caution patients to avoid alcoholic beverages and products containing aspirin or NSAIDs; may precipitate gastric bleeding.
- Instruct patient to notify health care professional immediately if symptoms of allergic reactions (rash, facial swelling, or difficulty breathing) or nausea, vomiting or diarrhea occur.
- May cause tiredness. Caution patient to avoid driving and other activities requiring alertness until response to medication is known.
- Advise patient this medication may have teratogenic effects. Contraception should be used by both men and women during and for at least 3 mo following completion of therapy. Advise women not to breastfeed during therapy.
- Instruct patient not to receive any vaccinations without advice of health care professional.
- Emphasize need for periodic lab tests to monitor for side effects.

Evaluation/Desired Outcomes

- Improvement in hematologic parameters.

---

bimatoprost (lash, ophthalmic)
(bi-**mat**-o-prost)
Latisse
Classification
Thera: hair regrowth stimulants
Pharm: prostaglandins

Pregnancy Category C

Indications

Treatment of eyelash hypotrichosis.

Action

Increases the percent of hair in eyelashes and prolongs the duration of growth phase. **Therapeutic Effects:** Increases eyelash growth, improving length, thickness and darkness.

Pharmacokinetics

Absorption: Minimal systemic absorption.
Distribution: Small amounts absorbed are widely distributed.
Metabolism and Excretion: Highly metabolized; 67% excreted in urine, 25% in feces mostly as metabolites.
Half-life: 45 min.

TIME/ACTION PROFILE (improvement in eyelash growth)

ROUTE	ONSET	PEAK	DURATION
Topical	2 mos	4 mos	4 wk or more*

*Following discontinuation.

Contraindications/Precautions

Contraindicated in: Hypersensitivity.
Use Cautiously in: Active intraocular inflammation; Patients with aphakia, pseudoaphakia with a torn posterior lens capsule, or know risk factors for macular edema; **OB:** Use in pregnancy only if potential benefit justifies potential risk to the fetus; **Lactation:** Use cautiously during lactation; **Pedi:** Safe and effective use in children has not been established.

Adverse Reactions/Side Effects

EENT: conjunctival hyperemia, eye pruritus, hyperpigmentation of eyelids, macular edema, permanent pigmentation of the iris.

Interactions

Drug-Drug: May ↓ the intraocular pressure lowering effect of **prostaglandin analogs**.

Route/Dosage

Topical (Adults): Apply to upper eyelid margin nightly.

Availability

Ophthalmic solution: 0.3 mg/mL provided as 3 mL in a 5 mL bottle.

NURSING IMPLICATIONS

Assessment

- Monitor intraocular pressure in patients with a history of increased intraocular pressure or who are using prostaglandin analogs for intraocular pressure reduction concurrently.

Potential Nursing Diagnoses

Disturbed body image (Indications)

Implementation

- **Topical:** Apply once each night using the accompanying sterile applicators. Additional applications will not increase the growth of eyelashes.

Patient/Family Teaching

- Instruct patient on correct application of bimatoprost. If a dose is missed, omit and apply next evening; do not double dose. Patient should wash face and remove all makeup and contact lenses prior to application. Contact lenses may be reinserted 15 min following administration. Place one drop of medication on the disposable sterile applicator and brush cautiously along the skin of the upper eyelid margin at the base of the eyelashes. Use only the applicator supplied with the product. Use each applicator for one eye then discard; reuse may result in contamination and infection. If solution gets into the eye, it is not harmful and does not need to be rinsed. Do not apply to lower lash line. Blot any excess solution outside upper eyelid margin with a tissue or other absorbent material. Do not allow tip of bottle or applicator to come in contact with surrounding structures, fingers, or any other unintended surface to avoid contamination. instruct patient to read the *Patient Information* guide prior to use and with each Rx refill, in case of new information.

- Inform patient that eyelid skin may darken with use of bimatoprost; may be reversible with discontinuation of medication. Instillation directly into eye may result in increased brown iris pigmentation; usually permanent.
- Inform patient of potential for hair growth occurring outside target treatment area if medication repeatedly touched same area of skin.
- Advise patient to notify health care professional immediately if eye trauma or infection, sudden decrease in visual acuity, conjunctivitis, or eyelid reactions occur or if having ocular surgery.
- Instruct patient to notify health care professional of bimatoprost use prior to intraocular pressure examinations.
- Advise female patients to notify health care professional if pregnancy is planned or suspected or if breastfeeding.

Evaluation/Desired Outcomes
- Increased length, thickness, and darkness or eyelashes. Onset is gradual and may not be noticed for 2 mos. Length, thickness, number of eyelashes, and/or direction of eyelash growth may vary between eyes. Upon discontinuation, eyelashes usually return to pretreatment level within 4 wks to mos.

C1 inhibitor (human)
(See-one in-**hib**-i-tor)
Cinryze

Classification
Thera: antiangioedema agents
Pharm: proteinase inhibitors

Pregnancy Category C

Indications
Routine prophylaxis against angioedema attacks in adult and adolescent patients with Hereditary Angioedema (HAE).

Action
Replaces C1 inhibitor which is deficient in patients with HAE. C1 inhibitor is necessary in preventing the chain of events which alter vascular permability resulting in life-threatening swelling in patients with HAE. **Therapeutic Effects:** Decreased frequency, intensity and duration of HAE attacks.

Pharmacokinetics
Absorption: IV administration results in complete bioavailibility.
Distribution: Unknown.
Metabolism and Excretion: Unknown.
Half-life: *Single dose*—56 hr.

TIME/ACTION PROFILE

ROUTE	ONSET	PEAK	DURATION
IV	within 1 hr	12 hr	3–4 days

Contraindications/Precautions
Contraindicated in: Life-threatening immediate hypersensitivity reactions. **Use Cautiously in:** Patients with known risk of thrombotic events; **OB: Lactation:** Use during pregnancy only if clearly needed; use cautiously during lactation; **Pedi:** Safe use in children, infants or neonates not established.

Adverse Reactions/Side Effects
CNS: headache. **Derm:** rash. **Misc:** Hypersensitivity reactions including ANAPHYLAXIS.

Interactions
Drug-Drug: None noted.

Route/Dosage
IV (Adults and adolescents): 1000 units every 3 or 4 days.

Availability
Powder for injections (requires reconstitution): 500 units/vial.

NURSING IMPLICATIONS

Assessment
● Assess for signs and symptoms of hypersensitivity reactions (hives, urticaria, tightness of the chest, wheezing, hypotension, anaphylaxis) during or after injection. Symptoms may be similar to HAE attacks; consider treatment methods carefully. If hypersensitivity occurs, discontinue infusion treat symptomatically. Epinephrine should be immediately available for treatment of acute severe hypersensitivity reaction.

● Monitor patients with known risk factors for thrombotic events.

Potential Nursing Diagnoses
Ineffective airway clearance (Indications)

Implementation
IV Administration

● **Intermittent Infusion: *Diluent:*** Reconstitute each of 2 vials with 5 mL of Sterile Water for Injection by removing the protective covering from one end of the double-ended transfer needle and inserting exposed needle through the center of the diluent vial stopper. Remove protective covering from the other end of the double-ended transfer needle. Invert diluent vial over the upright and slightly angled c1 inhibitor vial; then rapidly insert the free end of the needle through the center of the c1 inhibitor vial stopper. Vaccuum in the vial will draw in the diluent. Do not use if there is no vacuum

in the vial. Disconnect the two vials by removing the needle from the c1 inhibitor vial stopper and discard the diluent vial, along with the transfer needle directly into the sharps container. Gently swirl c1 inhibitor vial until all powder is completely dissolved. Solution is colorless to slightly blue; do not administer solutions that are discolored, turbid, or contain a precipitate. Insert the filter needle into the vial of reconstituted solution. Inject air into the vial and withdraw the reconstituted c1 inhibitor into the syringe. Repeat with a second vial to make complete dose. ***Concentration:*** 100 units/mL. Discard partially used vials. Attach a suitable needle or infusion set with winged adapter, and inject intravenously. Administer at room temperature within 3 hr of reconstitution. Do not freeze; protect solution from light. ***Rate:*** Administer at an initial infusion rate 1 mL/min over 10 min. If tolerated, continue same as the maintenance infusion rate.

● **Y-Site Incompatibility:** Do not mix with other materials.

Patient/Family Teaching
● Inform patient that c1 inhibitor is made from human plasma and may contain infectious agents that can cause disease.

● Instruct patient to notify health care professional immediately if signs and symptoms of allergic hypersensitivity reactions or thrombosis (new onset swelling and pain in limbs or abdomen, new onset chest pain, shortness of breath, loss of sensation or motor power, altered consciousness or speech) occur.

● Advise female patients to notify if health care professional if pregnancy is planned or suspected or if breastfeeding.

Evaluation/Desired Outcomes

- Decreased frequency, intensity and duration of HAE attacks.

---

certolizumab pegol
(ser-toe-**liz**-u-mab)
Cimzia

Classification
Thera: gastrointestinal anti-inflammatories—therapeutic
Pharm: tumor necrosis factor blockers

Pregnancy Category B

Indications
Moderately to severely active Crohn's disease when response to conventional therapy has been inadequate.

Action
Neutralizes tumor necrosis factor (TNF), a prime mediator of inflammation; pegolation provides a long duration of action. **Therapeutic Effects:** Decreased signs/symptoms of Crohn's disease.

Pharmacokinetics
Absorption: 80% absorbed following SC administration.
Distribution: Unknown.
Metabolism and Excretion: Unknown.
Half-life: 14 days.

TIME/ACTION PROFILE (blood levels)

ROUTE	ONSET	PEAK	DURATION
Subcut	unknown	50–120 hr	2–4 wk

Contraindications/Precautions
Contraindicated in: Active untreated infection; Hepatitis B reactivation; Concurrent use of anakinra.
Use Cautiously in: History of recurrent infections, concurrent immunosuppressants, medical conditions associated with increased risk of infection, current residence in areas where tuberculosis or histoplasmosis are endemic, history of hepatitis B infection (may reactivate); History of demyelinating disorders (may exacerbate); History of heart failure; **Geri:** May ↑ risk of infections; **OB:** Use in pregnancy only if clearly needed; avoid breastfeeding; **Pedi:** Safety not established.

Adverse Reactions/Side Effects
Derm: skin reactions (rarely severe).
Hemat: hematologic reactions. **MS:** arthralgia. **Misc:** allergic reactions including ANAPHYLAXIS, INFECTIONS (including reactivation tuberculosis and invasive fungal infections), MALIGNANCY, lupus-like syndrome.

Interactions
Drug-Drug: Concurrent use with **anakinra** ↑ risk of serious infections (contraindicated). May ↓ antibody response to or ↑ risk of adverse reactions to **live vaccines** (contraindicated).

Route/Dosage
Subcut: (Adults): 400 mg initially, repeat 2 and 4 wk later; may be followed by maintenance dose of 400 mg every 4 wk.

Availability
Lyophilized powder for subcutaneous injection (requires reconstitution): 200 mg vial, 100 mg vial.

NURSING IMPLICATIONS

Assessment
- Assess abdominal pain and frequency, quantity, and consistency of stools at beginning and during therapy.
- Assess for signs of infection (fever, sore throat, dyspnea, WBC) prior to and during therapy. Monitor all patients for active TB during therapy, even if initial test was negative. Do not begin certolizumab during an

active infection, including chronic or localized infections. If infection develops, monitor closely and discontinue certolizumab if infection becomes serious.

- Evaluate patients at risk for hepatitis B virus (HBV) infection for prior evidence of HBV infection before initiating therapy. Monitor carriers of HBV closely for clinical and lab signs of active HBV infection during and for several months following discontinuation of therapy. If HBV reactivation occurs, discontinue certolizumab and initiate antiviral therapy.
- Monitor for signs of hypersensitivity reactions (angioedema, dyspnea, hypotension, rash, serum sickness, urticaria). If reactions occur, discontinue certolizumab and treat symptomatically.
- *Lab Test Considerations:* May cause anemia, leukopenia, pancytopenia, and thrombocytopenia.
- May cause ↑ liver enzymes.
- May cause erroneously ↑ aPTT.

Potential Nursing Diagnoses
Risk for infection (Side Effects)

Implementation
- Perform test for latent TB. If positive, begin treatment for TB prior to starting certolizumab therapy.
- Bring medication to room temperature prior to reconstituting. Reconstitute 2 vials for each dose by adding 1 mL of Sterile Water for injection to each vial, using a 20-gauge needle, for a concentration of 200 mg/mL. Gently swirl so all powder comes into contact with sterile water; do not shake. Leave vials undisturbed for as long as 30 min to fully reconstitute. Solution is clear and colorless to pale yellow; do not

administer solutions that are discolored or contain particulate matter. Do not leave reconstituted solution at room temperature for >2 hr prior to injection. May be refrigerated for up to 24 hr prior to injection; do not freeze.
- **Subcut:** Bring solution to room temperature prior to injection. Using a new 20-gauge needle for each vial, withdraw reconstituted solution into 2 separate syringes each containing 1 mL (200 mg/mL) of certolizumab. Switch each 20-gauge needle to a 23-gauge needle and inject the full contents of each syringe subcut into separate sides of the abdomen or thigh.

Patient/Family Teaching
- Advise patient of potential benefits and risks of certolizumab. Advise patient to read the *Medication Guide* prior to starting therapy.
- Inform patient of risk of infection. Advise patient to notify health care professional if symptoms of infection (fever, cough, flu-like symptoms, or open cuts or sores), including TB or reactivation of HBV infection occur.
- Counsel patient about possible risk of lymphoma and other malignancies while receiving certolizumab.
- Advise patient to notify health care professional if signs of hypersensitivity reactions (rash, swollen face, difficulty breathing), or new or worsening medical conditions such as heart or neurological disease or autoimmune disorders occur and to report signs of bone marrow depression (bruising, bleeding, or persistent failure.
- Instruct patient to consult health care professional prior to taking any Rx, OTC, vitamins or herbal products.

- Advise patient to notify health care professional if pregnancy is planned or suspected or if breastfeeding.

Evaluation/Desired Outcomes

- Decrease in signs and symptoms of Crohn's disease.

---

ciclesonide (inhalation)
(si-**kless**-o-nide)
Alvesco
Classification
Thera: antiasthmatics
Pharm: corticosteroids (inhalation)

Pregnancy Category C

Indications

Maintenance treatment of asthma as preventive therapy in patients ≥12 yr. Not for acute treatment of bronchospasm.

Action

Potent, locally acting anti-inflammatory and immune modifier. **Therapeutic Effects:** Decreased frequency and severity of asthma attacks; improved asthma symptoms.

Pharmacokinetics

Absorption: Negligible oral bioavailability, action is primarily local.
Distribution: Unknown.
Metabolism and Excretion: Converted by esterases to des-ciclesonide, the active drug, which is subsequently metabolized by the liver. Some further metabolites may be pharmacologically active. Mostly eliminated in feces via biliary excretion; <20% of des-ciclesonide is excreted in urine.
Half-life: *Ciclesonide*—0.7 hr; *Des-ciclesonide*—6–7 hr;.

TIME/ACTION PROFILE (improvement in symptoms)

ROUTE	ONSET	PEAK	DURATION
Inhaln	within 24 hr	1–4 wk†	unknown

† Improvement in pulmonary function, decreased airway responsiveness may take longer.

Contraindications/Precautions

Contraindicated in: Hypersensitivity to ciclesonide or any other ingredients in the formulation; Acute asthma/status asthmaticus.
Use Cautiously in: Geri: Consider age-related decrease in cardiac, renal and hepatic function, concurrent disease state and drug therapy; consider lower initial dose; **OB:** ↓ dose may be sufficient; **Lactation:** Many corticosteroids enter breast milk, hypercorticism may be seen with ↑ maternal doses; **Pedi:** Safety and effectiveness in children <12 has not been established.

Adverse Reactions/Side Effects

CNS: <u>headache</u>. **EENT:** candida infection of mouth and pharynx, <u>nasal congestion</u>, <u>nasopharyngitis</u>, pharyngolaryngeal pain, cataracts, ↑ intraocular pressure. **Endo:** adrenal suppression (↑ dose, long term therapy), ↓ growth (children). **MS:** <u>arthralgia</u>, <u>back pain</u>, ↓ bone mineral density (↑ dose, long term therapy), <u>extremity pain</u>. **Misc:** worsening of infections.

Interactions

Drug-Drug: None noted.

Route/Dosage

Inhaln (Adults ≥ 12 yr): *Previous therapy with bronchodilators alone*—80 mcg twice daily, may be increased to 160 mcg twice daily; *Previous therapy with inhaled corticosteroids*—80 mcg twice daily, may be increased to 320 mcg twice daily; *Previ-*

ous therapy with oral corticosteroids—320 mcg twice daily.

Availability

Aerosol inhalation (contains HFA-134A as a propellant): 80 mcg/actuation in 6.1 g cannisters of 60 actuations, 160 mcg/actuation in 6.1 and 9.6 g cannisters of 60 and 120 actuations.

NURSING IMPLICATIONS

Assessment

- Monitor respiratory status and lung sounds. Pulmonary function tests may be assessed periodically during and for several months following a transfer from systemic to inhalation corticosteroids.
- Assess patients changing from systemic corticosteroids to inhalation corticosteroids for signs of adrenal insufficiency (anorexia, nausea, weakness, fatigue, hypotension, hypoglycemia) during initial therapy and periods of stress. If these signs appear, notify health care professional immediately; condition may be life-threatening.
- Monitor for withdrawal symptoms (fatigue, weakness, nausea, vomiting, hypotension, joint or muscular pain, lassitude, depression) during withdrawal from oral corticosteroids.
- Monitor growth rates in children receiving chronic therapy; lowest possible dose should be used.
- Monitor patients with a change in vision or with a history of increased intraocular pressure, glaucoma, or cataracts closely.
- ***Lab Test Considerations:*** Periodic adrenal function tests may be ordered to assess degree of hypothalamic-pituitary-adrenal (HPA) axis suppression in chronic therapy. Children and patients using higher

than recommended doses are at highest risk for HPA suppression.

Potential Nursing Diagnoses

Ineffective airway clearance (Indications)
Risk for infection (Side Effects)

Implementation

- When changing from oral to inhaled corticosteroids, taper oral dose slowly, no faster than prednisone 2.5 mg/day on a weekly basis, beginning after at least 1 wk of ciclesonide inhalation therapy.
- After the desired clinical effect has been obtained, attempts should be made to decrease dose to lowest amount required to control symptoms. Gradually decrease as long as desired effect is maintained. If symptoms return, dose may briefly return to starting dose.
- **Inhaln:** Allow at least 1 min between inhalations. Do not shake inhaler or use with spacer (See Appendix D.).
- If bronchospasm occurs right after ciclesonide dose, discontinue and administer short acting bronchodilator; notify health care professional.

Patient/Family Teaching

- Instruct patient to use inhaler at regular intervals as directed. If a dose is missed, omit and take next regularly scheduled dose. Advise patient not to increase dose or discontinue medication, even if feeling better, without consulting health care professional; gradual decrease is required. If asthma symptoms worsen, contact health care professional. Instruct patient to read *Patient Leaflet* before use.
- Advise patient to follow instructions supplied. Before first-time use or if inhaler has not been used for more than 10 days, prime unit by actuating

3 times prior to dose. Do not shake inhaler. When dose indicator display window shows a red zone, 20 inhalations are left and refill is required; discard when indicator shows zero. Do not use actuator with other medications. Clean mouthpiece weekly with a clean dry tissue; do not wash or put any part of the inhaler in water.

- Advise patients using inhalation corticosteroids and bronchodilator to use bronchodilator first and to allow 5 min to elapse before administering the corticosteroid, unless otherwise directed by health care professional.
- Advise patient that inhalation corticosteroids should not be used to treat an acute asthma attack but should be continued even if other inhalation agents are used.
- Instruct patient to notify health care professional if asthma worsens or if signs of adrenal insufficiency occur.
- Patients using inhalation corticosteroids to control asthma may require systemic corticosteroids for acute attacks. Advise patient to use regular peak flow monitoring to determine respiratory status.
- Advise patient to rinse mouth with water after treatment to decrease risk of developing local candidiasis.
- Caution patient to avoid smoking, known allergens, and other respiratory irritants.
- Advise patient to notify health care professional if sore throat or mouth occurs or if exposed to anyone with chicken pox or measles.
- Instruct patient to consult health care professional before taking other Rx, OTC, or herbal products.
- Advise female patients to notify health care professional if pregnancy is planned or suspected or if breastfeeding.

- Instruct patient whose systemic corticosteroids have been recently reduced or withdrawn to carry a warning card indicating the need for supplemental systemic corticosteroids in the event of stress or severe asthma attack unresponsive to bronchodilators.

Evaluation/Desired Outcomes
- Management of the symptoms of chronic asthma.
- Improvement in asthma symptoms. Maximum benefit may take 4 wks or longer.

clevidipine (kle-**vi**-di-peen)
Cleviprex

Classification
Thera: antihypertensives
Pharm: calcium channel blockers (dihydropyridine)

Indications
Reduction of blood pressure when oral therapy is not feasible/desirable.

Action
Inhibits calcium transport into vascular smooth muscle, resulting in inhibition of excitation-contraction coupling and subsequent contraction. Decreases systemic vascular resistance; does not reduce cardiac filling pressure (pre-load). Has no effect on venous capacitance vessels. **Therapeutic Effects:** Decreases blood pressure.

Pharmacokinetics
Absorption: IV administration results in complete bioavailibility.
Distribution: Unknown.
Protein Binding: >99.5%.
Metabolism and Excretion: Rapidly metabolized by esterases in plasma and tissue to inactive metabolites; metabolites are excreted in urine (63–74%) and feces (7–22%).

Half-life: *Initial phase*—1 min; *terminal phase*—15 min.

TIME/ACTION PROFILE

ROUTE	ONSET	PEAK	DURATION
IV	2–4 min	30 min*	end of infusion

*Time to target blood pressure.

Contraindications/Precautions
Contraindicated in: Hypersensitivity; Allergy to soybeans, eggs/egg products, defective lipid metabolism including pathologic hyperlipidemia, lipoid nephrosis or acute pancreatitis; severe aortic stenosis.
Use Cautiously in: Geri: Titrate dose cautiously, initiate therapy at low end of dose range; consider age-related decrease in hepatic, renal or cardiac function, concomitant diseases or other drug therapy; **OB:** Use only if maternal benefit outweighs potential risk to fetus; **Lactation:** Consider possible infant exposure; **Pedi:** Safety not established for patients <18 yr.

Adverse Reactions/Side Effects
CNS: headache. **CV:** CHF, hypotension, rebound hypertension, reflex tachycardia. **GI:** nausea, vomiting. **MS:** arthralgia.

Interactions
Drug-Drug: ↑ risk of excess hypotension with other **antihypertensives**. Does not protect against effects of abrupt **beta blocker** withdrawal.

Route/Dosage
IV (Adults): *Initial dose:* 1–2 mg/hr; *Dose titration:* Double dose every 90 sec initially; as blood pressure approaches goal, increase dose by less than doubling and lengthen the time between dose adjustments to every 5–10 min. Usual dose required is 4–6 mg/hour. Severe hypertensive patients may require higher doses with a maximum of 16 mg/hr or less. Doses up to

32 mg/hr have been used, but generally should not exceed 21 mg/hr in a 24 hr period due to lipid load.

Availability
Emulsion for injection 0.5 mg/ml: 50 ml vial, 100 ml vial. **Cost:** wholesale cost $145/50–mL vial, $290/100–mL vial.

NURSING IMPLICATIONS
Assessment
- Monitor blood pressure and heart rate during infusion, and until vital signs stabilize. Hypotension and reflex tachycardia may occur with rapid upward titration. Monitor patients receiving prolonged clevidipine infusions and who have not been transitioned to other antihypertensive therapies for the possibility of rebound hypertension for at least 8 hrs after infusion is stopped; additional adjustments may be needed.

Potential Nursing Diagnoses
Ineffective tissue perfusion (Indications)

Implementation
- Discontinue clevidipine or titrate downward during initiation of oral therapy; consider time to onset of the oral agent's effect. Continue blood pressure monitoring until desired effect is achieved.

IV Administration
- **Intermittent Infusion: *Diluent:*** Do not dilute. Invert vial gently several times before use to ensure emulsion uniformity prior to administration. Solution is milky white; inspect for particulate matter and discoloration. Commercially available standard plastic cannula may be used to administer the infusion. Administer via central line or peripheral line. Solution is in single-use vials; discard unused portion 4

hr after stopper puncture. Store in refrigerator; once emulsion reaches room temperature, stable for 2 mo, do not re-refrigerate. *Rate:* Initiate intravenous infusion at 1-2 mg/hr. Administer using an infusion device allowing calibrated infusion rates.

- **Y-Site Compatibility:** Water for Injection, USP, 0.9% NaCl, D5W, D5/0.9% NaCl, D5/LR, LR, 10% amino acid.
- **Y-Site Incompatibility:** Do not administer in the same line as other medications.

Patient/Family Teaching

- Inform patient of the rationale for use of clevidipine.
- Advise patients to contact a health care professional immediately if signs of a new hypertensive emergency (neurological symptoms, visual changes, evidence of CHF) occur.
- Advise female patients to notify health care professional if pregnancy is planned or suspected or if breastfeeding.
- Encourage patients with underlying hypertension to continue follow up care and to continue taking their oral antihypertensive medication(s) as directed.

Evaluation/Desired Outcomes

- Decrease in blood pressure.

desvenlafaxine
(des-ven-la-**fax**-een)
Pristiq

Classification
Thera: antidepressants
Pharm: selective serotonin and norepinephrine reuptake inhibitors—SSNRIs

Pregnancy Category C

Indications
Treatment of major depressive disorder, often in conjunction with psychotherapy.

Action
Inhibits serotonin and norepinephrine reuptake in the CNS. **Therapeutic Effects:** Decrease in depressive symptomatology, with fewer relapses/recurrences.

Pharmacokinetics
Absorption: 80% absorbed following oral administration.
Distribution: Enters breast milk.
Metabolism and Excretion: 55% metabolized by the liver, 45% excreted unchanged in urine.
Half-life: 10 hr.

TIME/ACTION PROFILE (blood levels)

ROUTE	ONSET	PEAK	DURATION
PO	unknown	7.5 hr	24 hr

Contraindications/Precautions
Contraindicated in: Hypersensitivity to venlafaxine or desvenlafaxine; Concurrent MAO inhibitors or within 14 days of stopping an MAO inhibitor; after desvenlafaxine is stopped wait 7 days until starting an MAO inhibitor; Should not be use concurrently with venlafaxine.
Use Cautiously in: Untreated cerebrovascular or cardiovascular disease, including untreated hypertension (control blood pressure before initiating therapy); Bipolar disorder (may activate mania/hypomania); History of increased intraocular pressure/angle-closure glaucoma; Renal impairment (consider modifications, dose should exceed 50 mg/day, especially in moderate to severe renal impairment); History of seizures or neurologic impairment; Hepatic impairment (dose should not exceed 100 mg/day); Histo-

ry of suicide attempt (may increase suicidal ideation during initiation or dose change, especially in children, adolescents, and young adults); **Geri:** Consider age-related decrease in renal function, decreased body mass, concurrent disease states and mediations; **OB:** Use in pregnancy or lactation only if maternal benefit outweighs fetal/infant risk; **Pedi:** Safety and effectiveness unknown.

Adverse Reactions/Side Effects

CNS: SEIZURES, <u>anxiety</u>, <u>dizziness</u>, <u>drowsiness</u>, <u>insomnia</u>, headache. **EENT:** ↑ intraocular pressure, mydriasis. **Resp:** eosinophilic pneumonia, interstitial lung disease. **CV:** hypertension. **GI:** ↓ appetite, <u>constipation</u>, <u>nausea</u>. **GU:** <u>male sexual dysfunction</u>. **Derm:** <u>sweating</u>. **F and E:** hyponatremia. **Hemat:** ↑ risk of bleeding. **Metab:** hypercholesterolema, hyperlipidemia. **Misc:** serotonin syndrome.

Interactions

Drug-Drug: Concurrent use with **MAO inhibitors** may result in serious and potentially fatal interactions; avoid within 14 days of stopping an MAO inhibitor; after desvenlafaxine is stopped wait 7 days until starting an MAO inhibitor. ↑ risk of bleeding with other **drugs that** ↑ **bleeding risk** including **anticoagulants**, **antithrombotics**, **platelet aggregation inhibitors**, and **NSAIDs**. Use cautiously with other **CNS-active drugs**, including **alcohol** and **sedative/hypnotics** or **drugs that affect the serotonergic system**; effects of combination are unknown.

Route/Dosage

PO (Adults): 50 mg once daily
Renal Impairment
PO (Adults): *Moderate renal impairment*—50 mg/day; *CCR <30 ml/min*—50 mg every other day.

Availability

Extended-release tablets: 50 mg, 100 mg.

NURSING IMPLICATIONS

Assessment

● Assess mental status and mood changes, especially during initial few months of therapy and during dose changes. Inform physician or other health care professional if patient demonstrates significant increase in signs of depression (depressed mood, loss of interest in usual activities, significant change in weight and/or appetite, insomnia or hypersomnia, psychomotor agitation or retardation, increased fatigue, feelings or guilt or worthlessness, slowed thinking or impaired concentration, suicide attempt or suicidal ideation).

● Assess suicidal tendencies, especially in early therapy. Restrict amount of drug available to patient.

● Monitor blood pressure before and periodically during therapy. Sustained hypertension may be dose related; decrease dose or discontinue therapy if this occurs.

● Monitor appetite and nutritional intake; weigh weekly. Report continued weight loss. Adjust diet as tolerated to support nutritional status.

● Assess for serotonin syndrome (mental changes [agitation, hallucinations, coma], autonomic instability [tachycardia, labile blood pressure, hyperthermia], neuromuscular aberations [hyper reflexia, incoordination], and/or GI symptoms [nausea, vomiting, diarrhea]), especially in patients taking other serotonergic drugs (SSRIs, SNRIs, triptans).

● *Lab Test Considerations:* May cause ↑ fasting serum total choles-

terol, LDL, cholesterol, and triglycerides.
- May cause transient proteinuria, not usually associated with ↑ BUN or creatinine.
- May cause hyponatremia.

Potential Nursing Diagnoses
Ineffective coping (Indications)
Risk for injury (Side Effects)

Implementation
- **PO:** Administer at the same time each day, with or without food. Tablets should be swallowed whole; do not crush, break, chew, or dissolve.

Patient/Family Teaching
- Instruct patient to take medication exactly as directed at the same time each day. Take missed doses as soon as possible unless almost time for next dose. Do not double doses or discontinue abruptly; gradually decreased before discontinuation.
- Advise patient, family and caregivers to look for suicidality, especially during early therapy or dose changes. Notify health care professional immediately if thoughts about suicide or dying, attempts to commit suicide, new or worse depression or anxiety, agitation or restlessness, panic attacks, insomnia, new or worse irritability, aggressiveness, acting on dangerous impulses, mania, or other changes in mood or behavior or if symptoms of serotonin syndrome occur.
- May cause drowsiness or dizziness. Caution patient to avoid driving or other activities requiring alertness until response to the drug is known.
- Caution patient to avoid taking alcohol or other CNS-depressant drugs during therapy and not to take other Rx, OTC, or herbal products without consulting health care professional.

- Instruct female patients to inform health care professional if pregnancy is planned or suspected or if breastfeeding.
- Instruct patient to notify health care professional if signs of allergy (rash, hives, swelling, difficulty breathing) occur.
- Emphasize the importance of follow-up exams to monitor progress. Encourage patient participation in psychotherapy.

Evaluation/Desired Outcomes
- Increased sense of well-being.
- Renewed interest in surroundings. Need for therapy should be periodically reassessed. Therapy is usually continued for several mo.

dexlansoprazole
(dex-lan-**soe**-pra-zole)
Kapidex

Classification
Thera: antiulcer agents
Pharm: proton-pump inhibitors

Indications
Healing/maintenance of healing of erosive esophagitis (EE). Tretment of heartburn from non-erosive gastroesopahageal reflux disease (GERD).

Action
Binds to an enzyme in the presence of acidic gastric pH, preventing the final transport of hydrogen ions into the gastric lumen. **Therapeutic Effects:** Diminished accumulation of acid in the gastric lumen, with lessened acid reflux.

Pharmacokinetics
Absorption: Well absorbed following oral administration.
Distribution: Unknown.
Protein Binding: 96–99%.

Metabolism and Excretion: Extensively metabolized by the liver (CYP2C19 and CYP3A4 enzyme systems are involved) patients who are poor metabolizers may have higher blood levels; no active metabolites. No renal elimination.
Half-life: 1–2 hr.

TIME/ACTION PROFILE (blood levels)

ROUTE	ONSET	PEAK*	DURATION
PO	unknown	1–2 hr (1st); 4–5 hr) 2nd)	24 hr

*Reflects effects of delayed release capsule.

Contraindications/Precautions
Contraindicated in: Hypersensitivity; Severe hepatic impairment; **Geri:** Avoid nursing.
Use Cautiously in: Moderate hepatic impairment (daily dose should not exceed 30 mg); Safe use in children <18 yr not established.

Adverse Reactions/Side Effects
GI: <u>abdominal pain</u>, <u>diarrhea</u>, flatulence, nausea, vomiting.

Interactions
Drug-Drug: ↓ levels of **atazanavir**; do not administer concurrently. May ↓ absorption of drugs requiring acid pH for absorption, including **amipicillin**, **digoxin**, **iron salts** and **ketoconazole**. May increase effect of **warfarin**.

Route/Dosage
PO (Adults): *Healing of EE*—60 mg once daily for up to 8 wk; *maintenance of healing of EE*—30 mg once daily for up to 6 mo; *GERD*—30 mg once daily for 4 wk.

Hepatic Impairment
PO (Adults): *Moderate hepatic impairment*—daily dose should not exceed 30 mg.

Availability
Delayed release capsules: 30 mg, 60 mg.

NURSING IMPLICATIONS

Assessment
- Assess patient routinely for epigastric or abdominal pain and for frank or occult blood in stool, emesis, or gastric aspirate.
- *Lab Test Considerations:* May cause abnormal liver function tests, including ↑ AST, ALT, and ↑ or ↓ serum bilirubin.
- May cause ↑ serum creatinine and BUN, ↑ blood glucose, and ↑ serum potassium levels.
- May cause ↓ platelet levels.
- May also cause ↑ gastrin and total protein levels.
- Monitor INR and prothrombin time in patients taking warfarin.

Potential Nursing Diagnoses
Acute pain (Indications)

Implementation
- **PO:** May be administered without regard to food. Swallow capsules whole or may be opened and sprinkled on 1 tbsp of applesauce and swallowed immediately for patients with difficulty swallowing.

Patient/Family Teaching
- Instruct patient to take medication as directed for the full course of therapy, even if feeling better. Take missed doses as soon as remembered.
- Advise patient to avoid alcohol, products containing aspirin or NSAIDs, and foods that may cause an increase in GI irritation.
- Advise patient to report onset of black, tarry stools; diarrhea; or abdominal pain to health care professional promptly.

- Advise female patients to notify health care professional if pregnancy is planned or suspected or if breastfeeding.
- Instruct patient to consult health care professional prior to taking other Rx, OTC, or herbal products.

Evaluation/Desired Outcomes

- Decrease in abdominal pain heartburn, gastric irritation and bleeding in patients with GERD; may require up to 4 wks of therapy.
- Healing in patients with erosive esophagitis; may require up to 8 wks of therapy for healing and 6 mo of therapy for maintenance.

---

diclofenac (topical patch)
(dye-**kloe**-fen-ak)
Flector

Classification
Thera: nonsteroidal anti-inflammatory agents, analgesics

Pregnancy Category C

Indications
Topical treatment of acute pain due to minor strains, sprains, and contusions.

Action
Inhibits prostaglandin synthesis. **Therapeutic Effects:** Decreased pain.

Pharmacokinetics
Absorption: Well absorbed following topical application.
Distribution: Unknown.
Protein Binding: >99%.
Metabolism and Excretion: Mostly metabolized by the liver, metabolites are excreted in urine and bile.
Half-life: 12 hr.

TIME/ACTION PROFILE

ROUTE	ONSET	PEAK	DURATION
Top	unknown	10–20 hr	unknown

Contraindications/Precautions
Contraindicated in: Hypersensitivity; cross-sensitivity with other NSAIDs may exist; History of Aspirin Triad (nasal polyps, asthma, bronchospasm following aspirin); Treatment of perioperative pain following coronary artery bypass graft (CABG) surgery; Advanced renal disease; Application to non-intact or damaged skin; **OB:** Late pregnancy (may cause premature closure of the ductus arteriosus) or lactation.

Use Cautiously in: Geri: Increased risk of adverse effects; consider age-related decrease in metabolic pathways, concurrent disease states and drug therapy; History of cardiovascular disease or risk factors (increased risk of serious cardiovascular effects); History of hypertension or edema (may exacerbate condition); History of impaired renal or hepatic function, heart failure, concurrent ACE inhibitor or diuretic therapy (increased risk of renal toxicity); Chronic corticosteroid therapy (slow tapering of corticosteroids required); Bleeding abnormalities or platelet dysfunction; **Pedi:** Safe use not established.

Exercise Extreme Caution in: History of ulcer disease or GI bleeding; Preexisting asthma.

Adverse Reactions/Side Effects
CV: edema, hypertension. **GI:** GI BLEEDING, ↑ liver enzymes. **GU:** renal toxicity. **Derm:** STEVENS-JOHNSON SYNDROME, TOXIC EPIDERMAL NECROLYSIS, local reactions at treatment site, rash. **Misc:** allergic reactions including ANAPHYLATOID REACTIONS.

Interactions
Drug-Drug: Concurrent use with **aspirin** or **warfarin** may ↑ risk of adverse GI reactions. May ↓ antihypertensive response to **thiazide diuretics**, **ACE inhibitors**, or **loop diuretics**. May ↑ blood levels and risk of

toxicity from **lithium** or **methotrexate**; careful monitoring required.

Route/Dosage
Topical (Adults): 1 patch applied to most painful area twice daily.

Availability
Topical patch: 180 mg/patch.

NURSING IMPLICATIONS

Assessment
- Patients who have asthma, aspirin-induced allergy, and nasal polyps are at increased risk for developing hypersensitivity reactions.
- Assess pain and limitation of movement; note type, location, and intensity before and 30–60 min after administration.
- Monitor blood pressure closely during initiation of treatment and periodically during therapy in patients with hypertension.
- *Lab Test Considerations:* Diclofenac has minimal effect on bleeding time and platelet aggregation.
- Monitor CBC and chemistry profile periodically during therapy. May cause anemia, liver or renal dysfunction.

Potential Nursing Diagnoses
Acute pain (Indications)

Implementation
- To minimize side effects, use the lowest effective dose for the shortest duration possible. Administration in higher than recommended doses does not provide increased effectiveness but may cause increased side effects.
- **Topical:** Apply patch to the most painful area twice a day. Do not apply to non-intact or damaged skin resulting from any etiology (exudative dermatitis, eczema, infected lesion, burns, wounds). Avoid contact with eyes; wash hands after applying, handling, or removing patch.

Patient/Family Teaching
- Instruct patient on correct application procedure for patch. Apply patch to most painful area. Change patch every 12 hr. Remove patch if irritation occurs. Fold used patches so adhesive sticks to itself and discard where children and pets cannot get them. Encourage patient to read the NSAID Medication Guide that accompanies the prescription.
- Instruct patients if patch begins to peel off to tape the edges. Do not wear patch during bathing or showering. Bathing should take place between scheduled patch removal and application.
- Caution patient to avoid concurrent use of alcohol, aspirin, acetaminophen, other NSAIDs, or other OTC medications without consulting health care professional.
- May cause serious side effects: CV (MI or stroke), GI (ulcers, bleeding), skin (exfoliative dermatitis, Stevens—Johnson Syndrome, toxic epidermal necrolysis) and hypersensitivity (anaphylaxis). May occur without warning symptoms. Advise patient to stop medication and notify health care professional immediately if symptoms of CV side effects (chest pain, shortness of breath, weakness, slurring of speech), GI side effects (epigastric pain, dyspepsia, melana, hematemesis), skin side effects (skin rash, blisters, fever, itching) or hypersensitivity reactions (difficulty breathing or swelling of face or throat) occur. Inform patient that risk for heart attack or stroke that can lead to death increases with longer use of NSAID medications and in people who have heart disease and that risk of ulcer increases

with concurrent use of corticosteroids and anticoagulants, longer use, smoking, drinking alcohol, older age, and having poor health.

- Instruct patient to notify health care professional of medication regimen before treatment or surgery.
- Advise patient to notify health care professional promptly if unexplained weight gain, swelling of arms and legs or hands and feet, nausea, fatigue, lethargy, pruritis, yellowing of skin or eyes, itching, stomach pain, vomiting blood, bloody or tarry stools, or flu-like symptoms, occur.
- Caution female patient to avoid use of diclofenac in last trimester of pregnancy and to notify health care professional if breastfeeding.
- Advise patient to minimize use of concurrent NSAIDs during transdermal therapy.

Evaluation/Desired Outcomes

- Decrease in severity of mild to moderate pain.

---

difluprednate (ophthalmic)
(dye-floo-**pred**-nate)
Durezol

Classification
Thera: ocular agents
Pharm: corticosteroids

Pregnancy Category C

Indications

Treatment of inflammation and pain associated with ocular surgery.

Action

Decreases inflammation. **Therapeutic Effects:** Decreased pain and inflammation following ocular surgery.

Pharmacokinetics

Absorption: Limited systemic absorption.

Distribution: Unknown.
Metabolism and Excretion: Unknown.
Half-life: Unknown.

TIME/ACTION PROFILE

ROUTE	ONSET	PEAK	DURATION
Ophth	unknown	unknown	unknown

Contraindications/Precautions

Contraindicated in: Active viral, mycobacterial or fungal infection of eyes and surrounding structures.
Use Cautiously in: OB: Use in pregnancy only if potential benefit justifies potential risk to the fetus; **Lactation:** Use cautiously during lactation; **Pedi:** Safety and effectiveness in children have not been established.

Adverse Reactions/Side Effects

EENT: ↑ intraocular pressure, blepharitis, cataracts, conjunctival hyperemia, corneal edema, delayed healing, eye pain, infections, iritis, photophobia.

Interactions

Drug-Drug: None noted.

Route/Dosage

Ophth (Adults): 1 drop four times daily, starting 24 hr after surgery for 2 wk, then twice daily for one week, then further tapered based on response.

Availability

Ophthamic emulsion: 0.05% in 5 mL bottle.

NURSING IMPLICATIONS

Assessment

- Assess affected eye for pain and swelling during therapy.
- Monitor intraocular pressure of difluprednate is used more than 10 days.

Potential Nursing Diagnoses

Acute pain (Indications)

Implementation Ophth: Instill 1 drop into conjunctival sac of affected eye 4 times/day beginning 24 hrs after surgery and continuing throughout first 2 wks of postoperative period, followed by twice daily for a wk, then base dose on patient response.

Patient/Family Teaching

- Instruct patient in correct technique and frequency for instillation of eye drops (see Appendix D.).
- Instruct patient to avoid wearing contact lenses during therapy.
- Advise female patients to notify health care professional if pregnancy is planned or suspected or if breastfeeding.
- Advise patient to notify health care professional if redness, itching or inflammation develops or becomes aggravated.

Evaluation/Desired Outcomes

- Decrease in eye pain and inflammation following ocular surgery.

---

doripenem (do-ri-**pen**-em)
Doribax
Classification
Thera: anti-infectives
Pharm: carbapenems

Pregnancy Category B

Indications

Infections caused by susceptible organisms including: complicated intra-abdominal infections, complicated urinary tract infections, including pyelonephritis.

Action

Inhibits bacterial cell wall formation. **Therapeutic Effects:** Bactericidal action against susceptible bacteria. **Spectrum:** Active against the following gram-negative organisms: *Acinetobacter baumanii*, *Escherichia coli*, *Klebsiella pneumonia*, *Proteus mirabilis*, and *Pseudomonas aeruginosa*. Also active against the following gram-positive organisms: *Streptococcus constellatus* and *Streptococcus intermedius*. Anaerobic spectrum includes *Bacteroides caccae*, *Bacteroides fragilis*, *Bacteroides thetaiotaomicron*, *Bacteroides uniformis*, *Bacteroides vulgatus*, and *Peptostreptococcus micros*.

Pharmacokinetics

Absorption: IV administration results in complete bioavailability.
Distribution: Penetrates renal and peritoneal and retroperitoneal tissues and fluids.
Metabolism and Excretion: Mostly excreted unchanged in urine; minimal metabolism.
Half-life: 1 hr.

TIME/ACTION PROFILE (blood levels)

ROUTE	ONSET	PEAK	DURATION
IV	unknown	end of infusion	8 hr*

*Normal renal function.

Contraindications/Precautions

Contraindicated in: Hypersensitivity to doripenem, other carbapenems or beta-lactams.
Use Cautiously in: Geri: Consider age-related decrease in renal function when choosing dose; **OB:** Use cautiously during lactation; **Pedi:** Safe use in children has not been established.

Adverse Reactions/Side Effects

CV: headache. **GI:** PSEUDOMEMBRANOUS COLITIS, diarrhea, nausea, ↑ liver enzymes. **Hemat:** anemia. **Local:** phlebitis. **Misc:** allergic reactions including ANAPHYLAXIS, infection with resistant organisms, superinfection.

Interactions
Drug-Drug: None noted.
Drug-Natural Products: May ↓ blood levels of **valproic acid**; this may result in loss of seizure control. **Probenecid** ↓ renal clearance and ↑ blood levels.

Route/Dosage
IV (Adults): 500 mg every 8 hr **Renal Impairment**
IV (Adults): *CCr 30–50 ml/min—* 250 mg every 8 hr; *CCr >10–<30 ml/ min—*250 mg every 12 hr.

Availability
Powder for injection (requires reconstitution): 500 mg/vial.

NURSING IMPLICATIONS

Assessment
- Assess patient for infection (vital signs; appearance of wound, sputum, urine, and stool; WBC) at beginning of and during therapy.
- Obtain a history before initiating therapy to determine previous use of and reactions to penicillins, cephalosporins or carbapenems. Persons with a negative history of penicillin sensitivity may still have an allergic response.
- Obtain specimens for culture and sensitivity before initiating therapy. First dose may be given before receiving results.
- Observe patient for signs and symptoms of anaphylaxis (rash, pruritus, laryngeal edema, wheezing). Discontinue the drug and notify the physician immediately if these occur. Have epinephrine, an antihistamine, and resuscitative equipment close by in the event of an anaphylactic reaction.
- *Lab Test Considerations:* May cause ↑ AST, ALT, serum alkaline phosphatase levels.
- May cause anemia.

Potential Nursing Diagnoses
Risk for infection (Indications, Side Effects)

Implementation
- May switch to appropriate oral therapy after at least 3 days of parenteral therapy, once clinical improvement has been demonstrated.

IV Administration
- **Intermittent Infusion:** Reconstitute 500-mg vial with 10 mL of sterile injection or 0.9% NaCl and shake gently to form a suspension of 50 mg/mL. *Diluent:* Withdraw the resulting solution using a 21–gauge needle and add it to 100 mL of 0.9% NaCl or D5W; gently shake until clear. *For moderate or severe renal impairment, withdraw 55 mL of this solution from the bag and discard.* Solution should be clear and colorless to slightly yellow. *Concentration:* Final concentration is 4.5 mg/mL. Suspension is stable for 1hr prior to dilution in infusion bag. Administer within 8 hr of reconstitution with 0.9% NaCl or 4 hrs of reconstitution with D5W at room temperature or 24 hr if refrigerated; do not freeze. *Rate:* Administer over 1 hr. Do not give direct IV.
- **Y-Site Incompatibility:** Do not mix with or physically add to solutions containing other medications.

Patient/Family Teaching
- Advise patient to report the signs of superinfection (black, furry overgrowth on the tongue; vaginal itching or discharge; loose or foul-smelling stools) and allergy. Consult health care professional before treating with antidiarrheals.
- Caution patient to notify health care professional if fever and diarrhea occur, especially if stool contains blood, pus, or mucus. Advise patient

not to treat diarrhea without consulting health care professional. May occur up to several wk after discontinuation of medication.

Evaluation/Desired Outcomes

- Resolution of the signs and symptoms of infection. Length of time for complete resolution depends on the organism and site of infection. Duration may be extended up to 14 days for patients with concurrent bacteremia.

---

eltrombopag
(el-**trom**-bo-pag)
Promacta

Classification
Thera: antithrombocytopenics
Pharm: thrombopoetin receptor agonists

Pregnancy Category C

Indications

Treatment of chronic immune (idiopathic) thrombocytopenic purpura in patients who have had an inadequate response to cortocosteroids, immunoglobulins or splenectomy.

Action

Increases platelet production by initiating proliferation and differentiation of megakaryocytes from bone marrow progenitor cells. **Therapeutic Effects:** Increased platelet count with reduced risk of bleeding.

Pharmacokinetics

Absorption: 52% absorbed following oral administration.
Distribution: Unknown.
Protein Binding: >99%.
Metabolism and Excretion: Extensively metabolized; 59% eliminated in feces, 20% as unchanged drug; 31% excreted in urine as metabolites.

Half-life: 21–35 hr.

TIME/ACTION PROFILE (effect on platelet count)

ROUTE	ONSET	PEAK	DURATION
PO	1 wk	2 wk	1 wk

Contraindications/Precautions

Contraindicated in: Lactation: Lactation.

Use Cautiously in: Myelodysplastic syndromes (may ↑ risk of hematologic malignancy); Hepatic impairment (lower initial dose may be required); Patients with East Asian ancestry (may require lower doses); **Geri:** Elderly patients may be more sensitive to drug effects; increase dose cautiously, consider age-related decrease in renal and hepatic function, concurrent disease states and drug therapy; **OB:** Use in pregnancy only when potential maternal benefit outweighs potential risk to fetus.

Adverse Reactions/Side Effects

EENT: development/worsening of cataracts. **GI:** HEPATOTOXICITY. **Hemat:** bone marrow changes.

Interactions

Drug-Drug: ↓ availability and absorption of **iron**, **calcium**, **aluminum**, **magnesium**, **selenium** and **zinc** by chelation; do not administer within 4 hr of medications containing these and other polyvalent cations.
Drug-Food: ↓ availability and absorption of **iron**, **calcium**, **aluminum**, **magnesium**, **selenium**, and **zinc** by chelation; do not administer within 4 hr of foods containing these and other polyvalent cations.

Route/Dosage

PO (Adults): 50 mg once daily, may be increased to achieve a platelet count of ≥50 × 10⁹/L (not to exceed 75 mg/

day); *patient of East Asian ancestry or moderate to severe hepatic impairment*— 25 mg once daily initially, may be increased to achieve a platelet count of ≥50 × 10⁹/L (not to exceed 75 mg/day).

Availability

Tablets: 25 mg, 50.

NURSING IMPLICATIONS

Assessment

- Monitor for unusual bleeding and bruising and signs of hepatotoxicity during therapy.
- Monitor for signs and symptoms of cataracts. Perform baseline ocular examination prior to administration and periodically during therapy.
- *Lab Test Considerations:* Modify dose based on platelet count. *If platelet count <50 × 10⁹/L following at least 2 wk of therapy,* increase daily dose by 25 mg. *If platelet count is ≥200 × 10⁹/L to ≤400 × 10⁹/L,* decrease dose by 25 mg. Wait 2 wk to assess effects of dose adjustment. *If platelet count >400 × 10⁹/L,* stop eltrombopag, increase monitoring of platelet monitoring to 2x/wk. Once platelet count is <150 × 10⁹/L, reinititate therapy at dose reduced by 25 mg/day. *If platelet count >400 × 10⁹/L after 2 wk of therapy at lowest dose,* permanently discontinue eltrombopag. Discontinue eltrombopag if platelet count does not ↑ to a level sufficient to avoid clinically important bleeding after 4 wk of therapy at maximum daily dose of 75 mg.
- Monitor liver tests and CBC, including platelet counts and peripheral blood smears, prior to and throughout therapy. Monitor AST, ALT, and serum bilirubin prior to therapy, every 2 wk during dose adjustment, and monthly following stable dose. If

bilirubin is ↑, perform fractionation. Evaluate abnormal liver tests with repeat testing in 3–5 days. If abnormalities are confirmed, monitor serum liver tests weekly until resolved, stabilize, or return to baseline. Discontinue eltrombopag if ALT levels ↑ to ≥3 × upper limit of normal and are progressive, persistent for ≥4 wk, or accompanied by ↑ direct bilirubin, or accompanied by clinical symptoms of liver injury or evidence of hepatic decompensation. Monitor CBC including platelet count, for at least 4 wk following discontinuation of therapy; may cause worsening thrombocytopenia.

Potential Nursing Diagnoses

Risk for injury (Adverse Reactions)

Implementation

- Available only through a restricted distribution program, *Promacta Cares*. ONly prescribers, pharmacies, and patients registered with the program are able to prescribe, dispense, and receive eltrombopag To enroll call 1-877-9-PROMACTA.
- **PO:** Administer on an empty stomach, 1 hr before or 2 hr after a meal. Allow at least 4 hr between eltrombopag and other medications (antacids), calcium-rich foods (dairy and calcium-fortified juices), and supplements containing iron, calcium, aluminum, magnesium, zinc, and selenium.

Patient/Family Teaching

- Explain purpose, risks and benefits of therapy to patient. Assist in enrollment in *Promacta Cares* program. Risks or long term therapy are unknown.
- Instruct patient to avoid taking eltrombopag within 4 hr of foods, mineral supplements, and antacids

containing iron, calcium, aluminum, magnesium, zinc, and selenium.
- Advise patients to avoid activities that may increase risk of bleeding.
- Instruct patient to notify health care professional if symptoms of liver problems (yellowing of skin or whites of eyes, unusual darkening of urine, unusual tiredness, pain in right upper stomach) occur.
- Advise female patients to notify health care professional promptly if pregnancy is planned or suspected or if breastfeeding. A pregnancy registry has been established to collect information about eltrombopag effects during pregnancy. Enrollment is by calling 1-888-825-5249.
- Emphasize the importance of routine lab tests to determine effectiveness and monitor for side effects.

Evaluation/Desired Outcomes
- Increased platelet counts and decreased risk of bleeding. Platelet counts usually increase within 1–2 wk of starting and decrease within 1–2 wk of discontinuing therapy.

---

etravirine (e-tra-*veer*-een)
Intelence
Classification
Thera: antiretrovirals
Pharm: non-nucleoside reverse transcriptase inhibitors

Pregnancy Category B

Indications
HIV infection (with other antiretrovirals).

Action
Binds to the enzyme reverse transcriptase which results in disrupted viral DNA synthesis. **Therapeutic Effects:** Evidence of decreased viral replication and reduced viral load with slowed progression of HIV and its sequelae.

Pharmacokinetics
Absorption: Well absorbed following oral administration. Food enhances absorption.
Distribution: Unknown.
Protein Binding: 99.9%.
Metabolism and Excretion: Mostly metabolized by the liver (CYP3A4, CYP2C9 and CYP2C19 enzyme systems); minimal renal excretion; mostly eliminated in feces as unchanged drug and metabolites.
Half-life: 41 hr.

TIME/ACTION PROFILE (blood levels)

ROUTE	ONSET	PEAK	DURATION
PO	unknown	2.5–4 hr	12 hr

Contraindications/Precautions
Contraindicated in: Concurrent use with other non-nucleoside reverse transcriptase inhibitors (NNRTIs), rifampin, rifapentine, St. John's wort.
Use Cautiously in: Concurrent use of antiarrhythmics, anticonvulsants, antifungals, clarithromycin, rifabutin, diazepam, dexamethasone, HMG CoA reductase inhibitors (statins), immunusuppressants; **Geri:** Consider age-related ↓ in organ function and body mass, concurrent disease states and medications; **Pedi, OB, Lactation:** Safety not established, breast-feeding not recommended in HIV-infected women.

Adverse Reactions/Side Effects
CNS: SEIZURES, anxiety, confusion, fatigue, headache, insomnia, sleep disorders. **EENT:** blurred vision, vertigo. **CV:** MYOCARDIAL INFARCTION, angina pectoris, atrial fibrillation, hypertension. **GI:** <u>nausea</u>, abdominal pain, anorexia, dry mouth, hepatitis, stomatitis, vomiting. **GU:** renal failure. **Endo:** gynecomastia, hyperglycemia, hyperlipidemia. **Hemat:** anemia, hemolytic anemia. **Derm:** <u>rash</u>. **Metab:**

fat redistribution. **Neuro:** peripheral neuropathy. **MS:** hemarthrosis. **Misc:** allergic reactions including STEVENS-JOHNSON SYNDROME, IMMUNE RECONSTITUTION SYNDROME.

Interactions

Drug-Drug: Etravirine is a substrate of the **CYP3A4**, **CYP2C9**, and **CYP2C19** enzyme systems; other medications the induce or inhibit these systems may be expected to alter the response to etravirine. Etravirine is an inducer of **CYP3A4** and an inhibitor of **CYP2C9** and **CYP2C19**. The effects of medications that are substrates of these enzyme systems may be altered by concurrent use. Concurrent use with other **NNRTIs** including **efavirenz**, **nevirapine**, and **delavirdine** may lead to ↓ effectiveness and should be avoided. Concurrent use with **protease inhibitors (PIs)** including **atazanavir**, **fosamprenavir**, **nelfinavir**, and **indinavir** may lead to altered plasma levels and should be undertaken with concurrent low dose **ritonavir**. Concurrent use with higher dose **ritonavir**, combination **tipranavir/ritonavir**, **fosamprenavir/ritonavir**, **atazanavir/ritonavir** alter levels and effectiveness of etravirine and should be avoided. Concurrent use of the combination **saquinavir/ritonavir** should be undertake cautiously. ↓ blood levels and effectiveness of **antiarrhythmics** including **amiodarone**, **bepridil**, **disopyramide**, **flecainide**, **lidocaine**, **mexiletine**, **quinidine**, **propafenone**, and **quinidine**; blood level monitoring recommended. Blood levels and effects may be ↓ by anticonvulsants including **carbamazepine**, **phenobarbital**, and **phenytoin**. Concurrent use with **voriconazole** may ↑ levels of both drugs; ↓ levels of **itraconazole** and **ketoconazole** (dose adjustments may be necessary).

May alter levels and response to **clarithromycin**; other agents should be considered. **Rifampin** and **rifapentine** ↓ blood levels and effectiveness and should be avoided; **rifabutin** should only be used without a protease inhibitor/ritonavir combination. May ↑ blood levels and sedation from **diazepam**, monitor for effects. Levels and effectiveness may be ↓ by **dexamethasone** use cautiously and consider alternatives. May alter blood levels and effects of **fluvastatin**, **lovastatin**, and **simvastatin** (dose adjustments may be necessary. May alter blood levels and effects of **cyclosporine**, **sirolimus**, and **tacrolimus**; careful monitoring required.

Drug-Natural Products: *St. John's wort* may ↓ blood levels and effectiveness; avoid concurrent use.

Route/Dosage
PO (Adults): 200 mg twice daily.

Availability
Tablets: 100 mg.

NURSING IMPLICATIONS

Assessment

- Assess for change in severity of HIV symptoms and for symptoms of opportunistic infections during therapy.
- Assess patient for rash (mild to moderate rash usually occurs in the 2nd wk of therapy and resolves within 1– 2 wk of continued therapy. If rash is severe (extensive erythematous or maculopapular rash with moist desquamation or angioedema) or accompanied by systemic symptoms (serum sickness-like reaction, Stevens–Johnson syndrome, toxic epidermal necrolysis), therapy must be discontinued immediately.
- *Lab Test Considerations:* Monitor viral load and CD4 cell count regularly during therapy.

- Monitor liver function tests periodically during therapy. May cause ↑ serum AST, ALT concentrations.
- May cause ↑ pancreatic amylase and lipase.
- May cause ↑ in total cholesterol, low density lipoprotein, serum triglyceride, and glucose levels.
- May cause ↑ serum creatinine.
- May cause ↓ neutrophils, ↓ platelet count, anemia and hemolytic anemia.

Potential Nursing Diagnoses
Risk for infection (Indications)
Noncompliance (Patient/Family Teaching)

Implementation
- **PO:** Administer 2 tablets twice daily following a meal; type of food does not matter. Swallow tablet whole, do not crush, break, or chew. If patient has difficulty swallowing, may disperse tablet in a glass of water. Once dispersed, patient should stir well and drink immediately; rinse glass with water and drink several times to ensure entire dose is consumed.

Patient/Family Teaching
- Emphasize the importance of taking etravirine as directed, at the same time each day. It must always be used in combination with other antiretroviral drugs. Do not take more than prescribed amount and do not stop taking without consulting health care professional. Take missed doses following a meal if remembered within 6 hrs of the time its usually taken, then return to regular schedule. If more than 6 hrs from time dose is usually taken, omit dose and resume dosing schedule; do not double doses.
- Instruct patient that etravirine should not be shared with others.

- Inform patient that etravirine does not cure AIDS or prevent associated or opportunistic infections. Etravirine does not reduce the risk of transmission of HIV to others through sexual contact or blood contamination. Caution patient to use a condom and to avoid sharing needles or donating blood to prevent spreading the AIDS virus to others. Advise patient that the long-term effects of etravirine are unknown at this time.
- May cause dizziness, impaired concentration, or drowsiness. Caution patient to avoid driving or other activities requiring alertness until response to medication is known.
- Instruct patient to notify health care professional immediately if rash or signs of Immune Reconstitution Syndrome (signs and symptoms of an infection) occur.
- Advise patient to avoid taking other Rx, OTC, vitamins, or herbal products, especially St. John's Wort, without consulting health care professional.
- Inform patient that changes in body fat (increased fat in upper back and neck, breast, and around back, chest, and stomach area, loss of fat from legs, arms, and face) may occur.
- Advise patients taking oral contraceptives to use a nonhormonal method of birth control during etravirine therapy and to notify health care professional if they become pregnant or plan to breastfeed while taking etravirine.
- Emphasize the importance of regular follow-up exams and blood counts to determine progress and monitor for side effects.

Evaluation/Desired Outcomes

- Delayed progression of AIDS and decreased opportunistic infections in patients with HIV.
- Decrease in viral load and increase in CD4 cell counts.

---

everolimus (e-ve-ro-li-mus)
Afinitor

Classification
Thera: antineoplastics
Pharm: kinase inhibitors

Pregnancy Category D

Indications

Advanced renal cell carcinoma which has failed treatment with sunitinib or sorafenib.

Action

Acts as a kinase inhibitor, decreasing cell proliferation. **Therapeutic Effects:** Decreased spread of renal cell carcinoma.

Pharmacokinetics

Absorption: Well absorbed following oral administration.
Distribution: 20% confined to plasma.
Metabolism and Excretion: Mostly metabolized by liver and other systems (CYP3A4 and PgP; metabolites are mostly excreted in feces [80%] and urine [5%]).
Half-life: 30 hr.

TIME/ACTION PROFILE (blood levels)

ROUTE	ONSET	PEAK	DURATION
PO	unknown	1–2 hr	24 hr

Contraindications/Precautions

Contraindicated in: Hypersensitivity to everolimus or other rapamycins; Severe hepatic impairment (Child-Pugh class C); **OB:** May cause fetal harm, avoid use during pregnancy; **Lactation:** Avoid breastfeeding.
Use Cautiously in: Moderate hepatic impairment (Child-Pugh class B); dose reduction required; **Geri:** Elderly patients may be more sensitive to drug effects; consider age-related decrease in hepatic function, concurrent disease states and drug therapy; **Pedi:** Safe use in children has not been established.

Adverse Reactions/Side Effects

CNS: <u>fatigue</u>, <u>weakness</u>, headache. **Resp:** PNEUMONITIS, <u>cough</u>, <u>dyspnea</u>. **GI:** <u>anorexia</u>, <u>diarrhea</u>, <u>mucositis</u>, <u>mouth ulcers</u>, <u>nausea</u>, <u>stomatitis</u>, <u>vomiting</u>, dysgeusia. **F and E:** peripheral edema. **Derm:** dry skin, pruritus, rash. **Hemat:** anemia, leukopenia, thrombocytopenia. **Metab:** hyperglycemia, hyperlipidemia, hypertriglyceridemia. **MS:** extremity pain. **Misc:** INFECTIONS, hypersensitivity reactions including ANAPHYLAXIS, fever.

Interactions

Drug-Drug: ↑ blood levels and risk of toxicity with **moderate and strong inhibitors of CYP 3A4 enzyme system and PgP** including **amprenavir, aprepitant, atazanvir, clarithromycin, delavirdine, diltiazem erythromycin, fluconazole fosamprenavir, indinavir, itraconazole ketoconazole, nefazodine, nelfinavir, ritonavir, saquinavir, telithromycin, verapamil** and **voriconazole**; avoid concurrent use. Avoid concurrent use with **CYP3A4 inducers** including **carbamazepine, dexamethasone, phenobarbital, phenytoin, rifabutin** and **rifampin**; ↑ dose of everolimus may be required. May ↓ antibody formation and ↑ risk of adverse reactions from **live virus vaccines**. ↑ blood levels and risk of toxicity with **grapefruit juice**; avoid concurrent use.

Route/Dosage
PO (Adults): 10 mg once daily; *Concurrent use of strong inducers of CYP3A4*— ↑ dose in 5 mg increments up to 20 mg/daily
Hepatic Impairment
PO (Adults): *Moderate hepatic impairment*—5 mg once daily.

Availability
Tablets: 5 mg, 10 mg.

NURSING IMPLICATIONS

Assessment
- Assess for symptoms of non-infectious pneumonitis (hypoxia, pleural effusion, cough, dyspnea) during therapy. If symptoms are mild, therapy may continue. Therapy should be interrupted for moderate symptoms and corticosteroids may be used. Re-initiate everolimus at a reduced dose of 5 mg/day when symptoms resolve.
- Assess for mouth ulcers, stomatitis, or oral mucositis. Topical treatments may be used; avoid peroxide-containing mouthwashes and antifungals unless fungal infection has been diagnosed.
- *Lab Test Considerations:* Monitor renal function prior to and periodically during therapy. May cause ↑ BUN and serum creatinine.
- Monitor fasting serum glucose and lipid profile prior to and periodically during therapy. May cause ↑ cholesterol, triglycerides, glucose. Attempt to achieve optimal glucose and lipid control prior to therapy.
- Monitor CBC prior to and periodically during therapy; may cause ↓ hemoglobin, lymphocytes, neutrophils, and platelets.
- May cause ↑ AST, ALT, phosphate, and bilirubin.

Potential Nursing Diagnoses
Risk for infection (Adverse Reactions)

Implementation
- **PO:** Administer without regard to food, followed by a whole glass of water. Tablets should be swallowed whole; do not break, crush, or chew. Avoid grapefruit juice and grapefruit products during therapy.

Patient/Family Teaching
- Instruct patient to take everolimus at the same time each day as directed. Take missed doses as soon as remembered up to 6 hr after time of normal dose. If more than 6 hr after normal dose, omit dose for that day and take next dose next day; do not take 2 doses to make up missed dose. Do not eat grapefruit or drink grapefruit juice during therapy. Advise patient to read *Patient Information Leaflet* prior to beginning therapy and with each Rx refill in case of new information.
- Advise patient to report worsening respiratory symptoms or signs of infection to health care professional promptly.
- Inform patient that mouth sores may occur. Consult health care professional for treatment if pain, discomfort, or open sores in mouth occur. May require special mouthwash or gel.
- Instruct patient to avoid use of live vaccines and close contact with those who have received live vaccines.
- Advise patient to consult health care professional before taking any Rx, OTC, or herbal products.
- May have teratogenic effects and decrease male and female fertility. Advise female patients to use effective contraception during and for up to 8

wks following therapy and to notify health care professional if pregnancy is planned or suspected or if breastfeeding.
- Emphasize the importance of routine blood tests to determine effectiveness and side effects.

Evaluation/Desired Outcomes
- Decreased spread of renal carcinoma. Continue treatment as long as clinical benefit is observed or until unacceptable toxicity occurs.

---

febuxostat (fe-**bux**-o-stat)
Uloric
Classification
Thera: antigout agents
Pharm: xanthine oxidase inhibitors

Pregnancy Category C

Indications
Chronic management of hyperuricemia in patients with a history of gout.

Action
Decreases production of uric acid by inhibiting xanthine oxidase. **Therapeutic Effects:** Lowering of serum uric acid levels with resultant decrease in gouty attacks.

Pharmacokinetics
Absorption: Well absorbed (49%) following oral administration.
Distribution: Unknown.
Protein Binding: 99.2%.
Metabolism and Excretion: Extensively metabolized by the liver; minimal renal excretion of unchanged drug, 45% eliminated in feces as unchanged drug, remainder is eliminated in urine and feces as inactive metabolites.
Half-life: 5–8 hr.

TIME/ACTION PROFILE (blood levels)

ROUTE	ONSET	PEAK	DURATION
PO	rapid	1–1.5 hr*	24 hr

*Maximum lowering of uric acid may take 2 wk.

Contraindications/Precautions
Contraindicated in: Concurrent azathioprine, mercaptopurine, or theophylline.
Use Cautiously in: Severe renal impairment (CCr <30 ml/min); Severe hepatic impairment; **OB:** Use in pregnancy only when potential maternal benefit outweighs potential fetal risk; **Pedi:** Safety in children <18 yr not established.

Adverse Reactions/Side Effects
GI: liver function abnormalities, nausea. **Derm:** rash. **MS:** gout flare, arthralgia.

Interactions
Drug-Drug: Significantly ↑ blood levels of, and risk of serious toxicity from, **azathioprine**, **mercaptopurine**, and **theophylline**; concurrent use is contraindicated.

Route/Dosage
PO (Adults): 40 mg once daily initially; if serum uric acid does not drop to <6 mg/dL dose should be increased to 80 mg daily.

Availability
Tablets: 40 mg, 80 mg.

NURSING IMPLICATIONS
Assessment
- Assess for joint pain and swelling, especially during early therapy. Changing serum uric acid levels from mobilization of urate from tissue deposits may cause gout flares. Use prophylactic NSAID or colchicine therapy for up to 6 months. If a gout flare occurs, continue febuxos-

tat therapy and treat flare concurrently.
- Monitor for signs and symptoms of MI and stroke.
- ***Lab Test Considerations:*** Monitor serum uric acid levels prior to, 2 wks after intitiating, and periodically thereafter. If serum uric acid levels are ≥6 mg/dL after 2 wks of daily 40 mg therapy, increase dose to 80 mg daily.
- Monitor liver function at 2 and 4 months of therapy and periodically thereafter. May cause ↑ AST, ALT, CPK, LDH, alkaline phosphatase and creatine.
- May cause prolonged aPTT and PT, and ↓ hematocrit, hemoglobin, RBC, platelet count, and lymphocyte, neutrohpil counts. May cause ↑ or ↓ WBC.
- May cause ↓ serum bicarbonate and ↑ serum sodium, glucose, potassium, and TSH levels.
- May cause ↑ serum cholesterol, triglycerides, amylase, and LDL levels.
- May cause ↑ BUN and serum creatinine and proteinuria.

Potential Nursing Diagnoses
Chronic pain (Indications)

Implementation
- **PO:** May be taken with or without food and with antacids.

Patient/Family Teaching
- Instruct patient to take febuxostat as directed. If a gout flare occurs, continue febuxostat and consult health care professional; medications to manage gout flare may be added.
- Advise patient to notify health care professional if rash, chest pain, shortness of breath, or stroke symptoms (weakness, headache, confusion, slurred speech) occur or if side effects are persistent or bothersome.

- Instruct patient to consult health care professional prior to taking any other Rx, OTC, or herbal products.
- Advise female patient to notify health care professional if pregnancy is planned or suspected or if breastfeeding.
- Emphasize the importance of follow up lab tests to monitor therapy.

Evaluation/Desired Outcomes
- Reduction in serum uric acid levels and resultant gout attacks.

---

fesoterodine
(fee-soe-**ter**-o-deen)
Toviaz
Classification
Thera: urinary tract antispasmodics
Pharm: anticholinergics

Pregnancy Category C

Indications
Treatment of overactive bladder function that results in urinary frequency, urgency, or urge incontinence.

Action
Acts as a competitive muscarinic receptor antagonist resulting in inhibition of cholinergically mediated bladder contraction. **Therapeutic Effects:** Decreased urinary frequency, urgency, and urge incontinence.

Pharmacokinetics
Absorption: Rapidly absorbed following oral administration, but is rapidly converted to its active metabolite (bioavailability of metabolite 52%; further metabolism occurs in the liver via CYP2D6 and CYP3A4 enzyme systems. 16% of active metabolite is excreted in urine, most of the remainder of inactive metabolites are renally excreted. 7% excreted in feces.

Distribution: Unknown.
Metabolism and Excretion: Rapidly converted by esterases to active metabolite.
Half-life: 7 hr (following oral administration).

TIME/ACTION PROFILE (active metabolite)

ROUTE	ONSET	PEAK	DURATION
PO	rapid	5 hr	24 hr

Contraindications/Precautions
Contraindicated in: Hypersensitivity; Urinary retention; Gastric retention; Severe hepatic impairment; Uncontrolled narrow-angle glaucoma.
Use Cautiously in: Significant bladder outlet obstruction (↑ risk of retention); Severe renal insufficiency (dose adjustment required); Decreased GI motility including severe constipation; Treated narrow-angle glaucoma (use only if benefits outweigh risks); Myasthenia gravis; Severe renal impairment (dose should not exceed 4 mg/day); **Geri:** ↑ risk of anticholinergic side effects in patients >75 yr; **OB: Lactation:** Avoid using unless potential benefits outweighs potential risk to fetus/neonate; **Pedi:** Safety in children not established.

Adverse Reactions/Side Effects
CV: tachycardia (dose related). **GI:** dry mouth, constipation, nausea, upper abdominal pain. **GU:** dysuria, urinary retention. **MS:** back pain.

Interactions
Drug-Drug: Concurrent use of **potent CYP3A4 enzyme inhibitors** including **ketoconazole**, **itraconazole**, and **clarithromycin** ↑ blood levels and risk of toxicity; daily dose should not exceed 4 mg. Use **less potent inhibitors of CYP3A4** (such as **erythromycin**) with caution; escalate dose carefully. Anticholinergic effects may alter the GI absorption of other drugs.

Route/Dosage
PO (Adults): 4 mg once daily initially may be increased to 8 mg/daily; *concurrent potent CYP3A4 inhibitors or CCr <30 ml/min*—dose should not exceed 4 mg/day.

Availability
Extended-release tablets: 4 mg, 8 mg.

NURSING IMPLICATIONS

Assessment
- Assess patient for urinary urgency, frequency, and urge incontinence periodically throughout therapy.
- *Lab Test Considerations:* May cause ↑ ALT and GGT.

Potential Nursing Diagnoses
Impaired urinary elimination (Indications)
Urinary retention (Indications)

Implementation
- **PO:** Administer without regard to food.
- Extended-release tablets should be swallowed whole; do not crush, break, or chew.

Patient/Family Teaching
- Instruct patient to take fesoterodine as directed. If a dose is missed, omit and begin taking again the next day; do not take 2 doses the same day. Advise patient to read the *Patient Information* sheet prior to initiation of therapy and with each Rx refill.
- May cause drowsiness and blurred vision. Caution patient to avoid driving or other activities requiring alertness until response to medication is known.
- Advise patient to avoid alcohol; may increase drowsiness.

- Advise patient to use caution in hot environments; may cause decreased sweating and severe heat illness.
- Instruct patient to consult health care professional before taking other Rx, OTC, or herbal products.
- Advise patient to notify health care professional if pregnancy is planned or suspected or if breastfeeding.

Evaluation/Desired Outcomes
- Decreased urinary frequency, urgency, and urge incontinence.

---

fosaprepitant (injection)
(fos-a-**prep**-i-tant)
Emend

Classification
Thera: antiemetics
Pharm: neurokinin antagonists

Pregnancy Category B

Indications
Prevention of nausea and vomiting associated with emetogenic chemotherapy.

Action
Acts as a selective antagonist at substance P/neurokinin$_1$ (NK1) receptors in the brain. **Therapeutic Effects:** Decreased nausea and vomiting associated with chemotherapy.

Pharmacokinetics
Absorption: Following IV administration, fosaprepitant is rapidly converted to aprepitant, the active component.
Distribution: Crosses the blood brain barrier; remainder of distribution unknown.
Metabolism and Excretion: Mostly metabolized by the liver (CYP3A4 enzyme system); not renally excreted.
Half-life: *Aprepitant*—9–13 hr.

TIME/ACTION PROFILE (antiemetic effect)

ROUTE	ONSET	PEAK	DURATION
PO	rapid	endo of infusion*	24 hr

* Blood level.

Contraindications/Precautions
Contraindicated in: Hypersensitivity; Concurrent use with pimozide (risk of life-threatening adverse cardiovascular reactions); **Lactation:** May cause unwanted effects in nursing infants. **Use Cautiously in: OB:** Use only if clearly needed; **Pedi:** Safety not established.

Adverse Reactions/Side Effects
CNS: dizziness, fatigue, weakness. **GI:** diarrhea. **Misc:** hiccups.

Interactions
Drug-Drug: Aprepitant inhibits, induces and is metabolized by the CYP3A4 enzyme system; it also induces the CYP2C9 system. Concurrent use with other medications that are metabolized by CYP3A4 may result in ↑ toxicity from these agents including **docetaxel**, **paclitaxel**, **etoposide**, **irinotecan**, **ifosfamide**, **imatinib**, **vinorelbine**, **vinblastine**, **vincristine**, **midazolam**, **triazolam**, and **alprazolam**; concurrent use should be undertaken with caution. Concurrent use with drugs that significantly inhibit the CYP3A4 enzyme system including **ketoconazole**, **itraconazole**, **nefazodone**, **clarithromycin**, **ritonavir**, **nelfinavir**, and **diltiazem** may ↑ blood levels and effects of aprepitant. Concurrent use with drugs that induce the CYP3A4 enzyme system including **rifampin**, **carbamazepine**, and **phenytoin** may ↓ blood levels and effects of aprepitant. ↑ blood levels and effects of **dexamethasone**, (regimen

reflects a 50% dose reduction); a similar effect occurs with **methylprednisolone** (IV dose by 25%, PO dose by 50% when used concurrently). May ↓ the effects of **warfarin** (careful monitoring for 2 wk recommended), **oral contraceptives** (use alternate method), **tolbutamide** and **phenytoin**.

Route/Dosage
IV (Adults): 115 mg 30 min prior to chemotherapy on day 1.

Availability
Lyophilized solid (requires reconsititution prior to injection): 115 mg/10–ml vial.

NURSING IMPLICATIONS

Assessment
- Assess nausea, vomiting, appetite, bowel sounds, and abdominal pain prior to and following administration.
- Monitor hydration, nutritional status, and intake and output. Patients with severe nausea and vomiting may require IV fluids in addition to antiemetics.
- *Lab Test Considerations:* Monitor clotting status closely during the 2 wk period, especially at 7–10 days, following fosaprepitant therapy in patients on chronic warfarin therapy.
- May cause mild, transient ↑ in alkaline phosphatase, AST, ALT, and BUN.
- May cause proteinuria, erythrocyturia, leukocyturia, hyperglycemia, hyponatremia, and ↑ leukocytes.
- May cause ↓ hemoglobin and WBC.

Potential Nursing Diagnoses
Risk for deficient fluid volume (Indications)
Imbalanced nutrition: less than body requirements (Indications)

Implementation
- Fosaprepitant is given as part of a regimen that includes a corticosteroid and a 5-HT₃ antagonist Administer dexamethasone 12 mg PO and ondansetron 32 mg IV 30 min prior to chemotherapy treatment on Day 1 of 3 day regimen.
- **Intermittent Infusion:** Inject 5 mL of 0.9% NaCl for Injection into vial. Swirl gently; avoid shaking or jetting saline into vial. *Diluent:* Prepare an infusion bag of 110 mL 0.9% NaCl. Withdraw entire volume from vial and transfer to infusion bag for a total volume of 115 mL. *Concentration:* 1 mg/mL. Gently invert bag 2–3 times. Solution is stable for 24 hr at room temperature. Inspect solution for particulate matter. Do not administer solutions that are discolored or contain particulate matter. *Rate:* Administer over 15 min.
- **Solution Incompatibility:** Incompatible with solutions containing divalent cations (calcium, magnesium) including LR and Hartmann's solution.

Patient/Family Teaching
- Instruct patient to notify health care professional if nausea and vomiting occur prior to administration.
- Advise patient to notify health care professional prior to taking any other Rx, OTC, or herbal products.
- Caution patient that fosaprepitant may decrease the effectiveness of oral contraceptives. Advise patient to use alternate nonhormonal methods of contraception during and for 1 mo following treatment.
- Advise patient to notify health care professional if pregnancy is planned or suspected or if breastfeeding.
- Advise patient and family to use general measures to decrease nausea (begin with sips of liquids and small,

nongreasy meals; provide oral hygiene; remove noxious stimuli from environment).

Evaluation/Desired Outcomes
- Decreased nausea and vomiting associated with chemotherapy.

---

fospropofol
(foss-**pro**-po-fol)
Lusedra
Classification
Thera: general anesthetics

Pregnancy Category B

Indications
Monitored anesthesia care (MAC) in adults undergoing diagnositic/therapeutic procedures.

Action
Mechanism of action is not known. **Therapeutic Effects:** Induction and maintenance of anesthesia.

Pharmacokinetics
Absorption: Fospropofol is a prodrug that is rapidly converted by enzymatic action to propofol, the active drug. IV administration results in rapid conversion.
Distribution: Propofol crosses the placenta and enters breast milk.
Protein Binding: 98%.
Metabolism and Excretion: Propofol is highly metabolized, neglagible renal excretion.
Half-life: *Fospropofol*—0.9 hr; *Propofol from fospropofol*—1.1 hr.

TIME/ACTION PROFILE

ROUTE	ONSET	PEAK*	DURATION
IV	rapid	8 min	5 min

*Peak effect meaning time to sedation and duration measuring time to fully alert.

Contraindications/Precautions
Contraindicated in: None noted.
Use Cautiously in: Compromised cardiac function, reduced vascular tone or reduced intravascular volume (↑ risk of hypotension); Hepatic impairment; Renal impairment (safety not established for CCr <30 ml/min); **Geri:** Patients ≥65 yr or those with severe systemic disease (dose reduction required); **OB: Lactation:** Not recommended for use during labor, delivery or lactation (may cause neonatal respiratory and cardiovascular depression); **Pedi:** Children <18 yr (safety not established, use not recommended).

Adverse Reactions/Side Effects
Resp: RESPIRATORY DEPRESSION, cough, hypoxemia. **CV:** hypotension. **Derm:** <u>pruritus</u>. **Neuro:** <u>paresthesia</u>. **Misc:** loss of purposeful responsiveness.

Interactions
Drug-Drug: May ↑ risk of cardio-respiratory depression when used with other **cardio-respiratory depressants** including **benzodiazepines** and **opioid analgesics**.

Route/Dosage
Patients weighing >90 kg should be dosed as if they are 90 kg; patients weighing <60 kg should be dosed as if they are 60 kg.
IV (Adults): 6.5 mg/kg (not to exceed 16.5 mL) initially, followed by supplemental doses of 1.6 mg/kg (not to exceed 4 mL or more frequently that every 4 min) as needed.

Route/Dosage
IV (Geriatric Patients ≥65 yr or those with severe systemic disease): 75% of standard dose.

Availability
Solution for injection: 1050 mg/30 mL.

NURSING IMPLICATIONS

Assessment

- Assess respiratory status, pulse, and blood pressure continuously throughout fospropofol therapy. May cause apnea. Use supplemental O_2 for all patients receiving fospropofol. Fospropofol should be used only by individuals experienced in endotracheal intubation, and equipment for this procedure should be readily available.
- Assess level of sedation and level of consciousness throughout and following administration.
- **_Toxicity and Overdose:_** If overdose occurs, monitor pulse, respiration, and blood pressure continuously. Maintain patent airway and assist ventilation as needed. If hypotension occurs, treatment includes IV fluids, repositioning, and vasopressors.

Potential Nursing Diagnoses

Ineffective breathing pattern (Adverse Reactions)
Risk for injury (Side Effects)

Implementation

- Dose is titrated to patient response. Administer supplemental doses based on level of sedation and level of sedation required for procedure; only when patient demonstrates purposeful movement in response to verbal or light tactile stimulation and no more frequently than every 4 min.
- Fospropofol has no effect on the pain threshold. Adequate analgesia should *always* be used when fospropofol is used as an adjunct to surgical procedures.

IV Administration

- **Direct IV: _Diluent:_** Administer undiluted. Shake well before use. Solution is clear and colorless; do not administer solutions that are discol-

ored or contain a precipitate. Contains no preservatives; maintain sterile technique and administer immediately after preparation. **_Concentration:_** Undiluted: 35mg/mL.

- Discard unused portions and IV lines at the end of anesthetic procedure. **_Rate:_** Administer over 3–5 min through a free-flowing IV line. Titrate to desired level of sedation. Flush line with 0.9% NaCl before and after administration.
- **Solution Compatibility:** D5W, 0.9% NaCl, 0.45% NaCl, LR, D5/LR, D5/0.45% NaCl, D5/0.2% NaCl, D5/0.45% NaCl with 20 mEq KClDo not mix with other drugs or fluids prior to administration.
- **Y-Site Incompatibility:** meperidine, midazolam.

Patient/Family Teaching

- Inform patient that this medication will decrease mental recall of the procedure.
- Inform patient that paresthesia (burning, tingling, stinging) and pruritus in the perineal region may occur upon injection of fospropofol; usually mild to moderate intensity, last a short time, and require no treatment.
- May cause drowsiness or dizziness. Advise patient to request assistance prior to ambulation and transfer and to avoid driving or other activities requiring alertness for 24 hr following administration.
- Advise patient to avoid alcohol or other CNS depressants without the advice of a health care professional for 24 hr following administration.

Evaluation/Desired Outcomes

- Induction and maintenance of anesthesia.
- Amnesia.
- Sedation in mechanically ventilated patients in an intensive care setting.

granisetron (transdermal)
(gra-**nees**-e-tron)
Sancuso

Classification
Thera: antianemics
Pharm: 5-HT$_3$ antagonists

Pregnancy Category C

Indications
Prevention of nausea and vomiting due to moderately/highly emetogenic chemotherapy.

Action
Blocks the effects of serotonin at receptor sites (selective antagonist) located in vagal nerve terminals and in the chemoreceptor trigger zone in the CNS.
Therapeutic Effects: Decreased incidence and severity of nausea and vomiting following emetogenic chemotherapy.

Pharmacokinetics
Absorption: Enters systemic circulation via passive diffusion through intact skin.
Distribution: Distributes freely between plasma and red blood cells.
Metabolism and Excretion: Mostly metabolized by the liver; 12% excreted unchanged in urine.
Half-life: *Patients with cancer*—8–9 hr (range 0.9–31.1 hr); *healthy volunteers*—4.9 hr (range 0.9–15.2 hr); *geriatric patients*—7.7 hr (range 2.6–17.7 hr).

TIME/ACTION PROFILE (blood levels)

ROUTE	ONSET	PEAK	DURATION
TD	unknown	48 hr	unknown

Contraindications/Precautions
Contraindicated in: Hypersensitivity.
Use Cautiously in: Underlying gastrointestinal pathology (may mask ileus/gastric distention; **Geri:** Consider age-related decrease in renal, hepatic or cardiac function, concurrent diseases and drug therapy; **OB, Lactation:** Use during pregnancy only if needed, use cautiously during lactation; **Pedi:** Safe use in children <18 yr not established.

Adverse Reactions/Side Effects
GI: constipation. **Derm:** application site reactions, photosensitivity.

Interactions
Drug-Drug: None reported.

Route/Dosage
PO (Adults): One 34.3 mg patch (delivers 3.1 mg/24 hr) applied up to 48 hr prior to chemotherapy, leave in place for at least 24 hr following chemotherapy, may be left in place for a total of 7 days.

Availability
Transdermal system (patch): Each patch contains 34.3 mg/52 cm^2 (delivers 3.1 mg/24 hr).

NURSING IMPLICATIONS
Assessment
- Assess patient for nausea, vomiting, abdominal distention, and bowel sounds prior to during, and following administration.
- Monitor application site. If allergic, erythematous, macular, or papular rash or pruritus occurs, remove patch.
- *Lab Test Considerations:* May cause ↑ AST and ALT levels.

Potential Nursing Diagnoses
Imbalanced nutrition: less than body requirements (Indications)

Implementation
- Remove patch prior to entering MRI.
- **Transdermal:** Apply system clear, dry, intact healthy skin on upper outer arm 24–48 hrs before chemo-

therapy. Do not use creams, lotions, or oils that may keep patch from sticking. Do not apply to skin that is red, irritated, or damaged. Apply immediately after removing from package. Do not cut patch into pieces. Remove liner from adhesive layer and press firmly in place with palm of hand for 30 sec, especially around the edges, to make sure contact is complete. Patch should be worn throughout chemotherapy. If patch does not stick, bandages or medical adhesive tape may be applied on edges of patch; do not cover patch with tape or bandages or wrap completely around arm. Patient may shower and wash normally while wearing patch; avoid swimming, strenuous exercise, sauna, or whirlpool during patch use. Remove patch gently at least 24 hrs after completion of chemotherapy; may be worn for up to 7 days. Fold so that adhesive edges are together. Throw away in garbage out of reach of children and pets on removal. Do not reuse patch. Use soap and water to remove remaining adhesive; do not use alcohol or acetone.

Patient/Family Teaching

● Instruct patient on correct application, removal, and disposal of patch. Advise patient to read *Patient Information* sheet prior to using and with each Rx refill in case of new information. Inform patient that additional granisetron should not be taken during patch application unless directed by health care professional.

● Instruct patient to remove patch when undergoing MRI examination.

● Advise patient to cover patch application site with clothing to avoid exposure to sunlight, sunlamp, or tanning beds during and for 10 days following removal of patch.

● May cause dizziness and drowsiness. Caution patient to avoid driving and other activities requiring alertness until response to medication is known.

● Instruct patient to notify health care professional if pain or swelling in the abdomen occurs or if redness at patch removal site remains for more than 3 days.

● Advise patient to consult health care professional prior to taking any other Rx, OTC, or herbal products.

● Advise female patient to notify health care professional if pregnancy is planned or suspected or if breastfeeding.

Evaluation/Desired Outcomes

● Prevention of nausea and vomiting associated with emetogenic cancer chemotherapy.

---

ixabepilone
(icks-a-**bep**-i-lone)
Ixempra
Classification
Thera: antineoplastics
Pharm: epothilone B analog

Pregnancy Category D

Indications

Combination use with capecitabine for the treatment of metastatic or locally advanced breast cancer currently resistant to a taxane and anthracycline or resistant to a taxane and cannot tolerate further anthracycline. May also be used as monotherapy for breast cancers that are not responding to anthracylines, taxane or capecitabine.

Action

Binds to β-tubulin subunits on microtubules; this action blocks cells in mitosis, leading to cell death. Also has antiangiogenic activity. **Therapeutic Ef-**

fects: Decreased spread of breast cancer.

Pharmacokinetics

Absorption: IV administration results in complete bioavailablity.

Distribution: Unknown.

Metabolism and Excretion: Extensively metabolized by the liver, primarily by the CYP3A4 enzyme system Metabolites are not active and are excreted mainly by the kidneys.

Half-life: 52 hr.

TIME/ACTION PROFILE (blood levels)

ROUTE	ONSET	PEAK	DURATION
IV	unknown	end of infusion	unknown

Contraindications/Precautions

Contraindicated in: Previous hypersensitivity to any medications containing Cremophor EL or similar derivatives (polyoxethylated castor oil); Neutrophils <1500 cells/m³ or platelets <100,000 cells/m³; Severe hepatic impairment; Use with capecitabine is contraindicated for hepatic impairment (AST or ALT >2.5 × upper limits of normal or bilirubin >1 × upper limit of normal) due to ↑ risk of toxicity and death associated with neutropenia; **OB:** Pregnancy or lactation.

Use Cautiously in: Toxicity; dose adjustments may be required for neuropathy/arthralgia/myalgia/fatigue, neutropenia, thrombocytopenia, moderate hepatic impairment or palmar-plantar erythrodysesthesia; Diluent contains dehydrated alcohol; consider possible CNS effects; Diabetes or history of neuropathy (↑ risk of severe neuropathy); History of cardiac disease (may ↑ risk of myocardial ischemia or ventricular dysfunction; **OB:** Patients with child-bearing potential.

Adverse Reactions/Side Effects

CNS: <u>fatigue</u>, <u>weakness</u>, dizziness, headache, insomnia. **EENT:** ↑ lacrimation. **CV:** chest pain, edema, myocardial ischemia, ventricular dysfunction. **Resp:** dyspnea. **GI:** <u>abdominal pain</u>, <u>anorexia*</u>, <u>constipation</u>, <u>diarrhea</u>, <u>mucositis</u>, <u>nausea</u>, <u>stomatitis</u>, vomiting, altered taste. **Derm:** <u>alopecia</u>, <u>hyperpigmentation</u>, <u>nail disorder</u>, <u>palmar-plantar erythrodysesthesia (combination therapy with capecitabine)</u>, exfoliation, pruritus, rash, hot flushes. **Hemat:** <u>MYELOSUPPRESSION</u>. **MS:** <u>arthralgia</u>, <u>musculoskeletal pain</u>, <u>myalgia</u>. **Neuro:** <u>peripheral neuropathy</u>. **Misc:** hypersensitivity reactions.

Interactions

Drug-Drug: **Strong CYP3A4 inhibitors** including **ketoconazole, itraconazole, voriconazole, clarithromycin, telithromycin, atazanavir, dalavirdine, ritonavir, saquinavir, nefazodone** ↑ blood levels and the risk of serious toxicities, concurrent use should be avoided if possible. If concurrent use is required, dose reduction of ixabepilone is recommended. Inducers of the **CYP3A4 enzyme system** including **dexamathasone, phenytoin, carbamazepine, phenobarbital, rifampin, rifampicin,** or **rifabutin** may ↓ levels and effectiveness, avoid if possible.

Drug-Natural Products: *St. John's wort* may ↓ blood levels and should be avoided.

Drug-Food: **Grapefruit juice** may ↑ blood levels and toxicity; avoid concurrent use.

Route/Dosage

IV (Adults): 40 mg/m² every 3 wk; not to exceed dose greater than that calculated for 2.2 m² (88 mg/dose)

Hepatic Impairment

IV (Adults): *Moderate Impairment*—20 mg/m² every 3 wk; not to exceed 30 mg/m².

Availability

Powder for injection (requires specific diluent for initial reconstitution): 15 mg vial (contains 16 mg ixebepilone to allow for withdrawal losses) with 8 mL of diluent in a separate vial as a kit, 45 mg vial (contains 47 mg ixebepilone to allow for withdrawal losses) with 23.5 mL of diluent in a separate vial.

NURSING IMPLICATIONS

Assessment

- Monitor for hypersensitivity reaction (flushing, rash, dyspnea, bronchospasm). If severe reactions occur stop infusion and provide aggressive supportive treatment with epinephrine and corticosteroids. In subsequent cycles, add corticosteroids to the premedication regimen.
- Monitor for myelosuppression frequently during therapy. Assess for signs of infection during neutropenia. Assess for bleeding (bleeding gums, bruising, petechiae, blood in stools, urine, and emesis) and avoid IM injections and taking rectal temperatures if platelet count is low. Apply pressure to venipuncture sites for 10 min.
- Assess patient for signs of peripheral neuropathy (burning sensation, hyperesthesia, hypoesthesia, paresthesia, discomfort, neuropathic pain); may occur early during treatment within the first 3 cycles. Patients experiencing new or worsening symptoms may require a reduction or delay in dose of ixabepilone. If neuropathy is Grade 2 (moderate) lasting for ≥7 days or Grade 3 (severe) lasting for <7 days decrease dose by 20%. If neuropathy is Grade 3 lasting ≥7 days or is disabling discontinue treatment.

- *Lab Test Considerations:* Monitor CBC and platelets frequently during therapy. If neutrophil count is <500 cells/mm^3 for ≥7 days or patient has febrile neutropenia or if platelet count is <25,000/mm^3 or platelets are <50,000/mm^3 with bleeding decrease the dose by 20%. Begin new treatment cycle only if neutrophil count is at least 1500 cells/mm^3 and nonhematologic toxicities have improved to Grade 1 (mild) or resolved. May also cause leukopenia and anemia.
- Monitor hepatic function prior to therapy. Patients with decreased hepatic function require a decreased dose. If AST and ALT ≤2.5 × the upper limits of normal (ULN) and bilirubin ≤1 × ULN administer ixabepilone at 40 mg/m^2. If AST and ALT ≤10 × the upper limits of normal (ULN) and bilirubin ≤1 × ULN administer ixabepilone at 32mg/m^2. If AST and ALT ≤10 × the upper limits of normal (ULN) and bilirubin >1.5 × ULN—≤3 × ULN administer ixabepilone at 20–30 mg/m^2.

Potential Nursing Diagnoses

Risk for injury (Adverse Reactions)

Implementation

- Premedicate patient with an H$_1$ and an H$_2$ antagonist approximately 1 hr before ixabepilone infusion. Patients who experienced a hypersensitivity reaction in a previous ixabepilone cycle should also be premedicated with corticosteroids and extension of the infusion time should be considered.
- To minimize risk of dermal exposure, wear impervious gloves when handling ixabepilone vials regardless of setting (unpacking and inspection, transport within a facility, dose preparation and administration).

IV Administration

- **Intermittent Infusion:** Remove *Ixempra kit* (containing ixabepilone vial and diluent vial) from refrigerator and allow to stand at room temperature for 30 min prior to diluting. *Ixempra kit* must be stored in refrigerator. When vials are first removed from refrigerator, a white precipitate may be observed in the diluent vial; precipitate will dissolve to form a clear solution once diluent warms to room temperature. **Diluent:** Use only diluent supplied in kit for reconstitution. Reconstitute 15–mg vial with 8 mL and 45–mg vial with 23.5 mL of diluent. Gently swirl and invert vial until powder is completely dissolved. Prior to administration, dilute constituted solution further with only LR supplied in DEHP free bags. Dilute as soon as possible after constitution, but may be stored at room temperature and room light for up to 1 hr. For most doses use 250 mL bag of LR. **Concentration:** If final concentration is not between 0.2 mg/mL and 0.6 mg/mL add to appropriate size bag of LR. Thoroughly mix infusion bag by manual rotation. Diluted solution is stable for up to 6 hr at room temperature and room light; must complete infusion during 6-hr period. Administer through an in-line filter with a microporous membrane of 0.2–1.2 microns. DEHP-free infusion containers and administration sets must be used. Discard remaining solution. **Rate:** Infuse over 3 hr.

Patient/Family Teaching

- Advise patient to avoid grapefruit juice during therapy; may lead to increased levels and side effects.
- Solution contains alcohol and may cause drowsiness or dizziness. Caution patient to avoid driving and other activities requiring alertness until response to medication is known.
- Instruct patient to notify health care professional promptly if fever >100.5°F; chills; cough; hoarseness; sore throat; signs of infection; lower back or side pain; burning, painful or difficulty urination; bleeding gums; bruising; petechiae; blood in stools, urine, or emesis; increased fatigue; dyspnea; or orthostatic hypotension occurs. Caution patient to avoid crowds and persons with known infections. Instruct patients to use a soft toothbrush and electric razor and to avoid falls. Caution patient not to drink alcoholic beverages or take medication containing aspirin or NSAIDs; may precipitate bleeding.
- Instruct patient to notify health care professional promptly if signs and symptoms of hypersensitivity (hives, urticaria, pruritus, rash, flushing, swelling, dyspnea, chest tightness), peripheral neuropathy (numbness and tingling in hands and feet), or cardiac adverse reactions (chest pain, difficulty breathing, palpitations, unusual weight gain) occur.
- Advise patient to consult health care professional before taking any Rx, OTC, herbal, or vitamin products, especially St. John's Wort, during therapy.
- Instruct patient not to receive any vaccinations without advice of health care professional.
- Discuss the possibility of hair loss with patient. Explore methods of coping. Regrowth usually occurs 2–3 mo after discontinuation of therapy.
- Advise women of childbearing potential to use effective contraception during therapy and to avoid breastfeeding during therapy.

Evaluation/Desired Outcomes
- Decreased progression of breast cancer.

---

lacosamide
(la-**kose**-a-mide)
Vimpat
Classification
Thera: anticonvulsants

Pregnancy Category C

Indications
Adjunctive therapy of partial-onset seizures.

Action
Mechanism is not known, but may involve enhancement of slow inactivation of sodium channels with resultant membrane stabilization also binds to collapsin response mediator protein-2 (CRMP-2) which is involved in neural differentiation and growth. **Therapeutic Effects:** Decreased incidence and severity of partial-onset seizures.

Pharmacokinetics
Absorption: 100% absorbed following oral administration; IV administration results in complete bioavailability.
Distribution: Unknown.
Metabolism and Excretion: Partially metabolized by the liver; 40% excreted in urine as unchanged drug, 30% as a metabolite.
Half-life: 13 hr.

TIME/ACTION PROFILE (blood levels)

ROUTE	ONSET	PEAK	DURATION
PO	unknown	1–4 hr	12 hr
IV	unknown	end of infusion	12 hr

Contraindications/Precautions
Contraindicated in: Hypersensitivity; Severe hepatic impairment; **Lactation:** Avoid use during breast feeding.

Use Cautiously in: CCr <30 ml/min (use lower daily dose); Mild to moderate hepatic impairment; titrate dose carefully, use lower daily dose; Known cardiac conduction problems or severe cardiac disease (MI or CHF); History of suicidal ideation or suicide attempt; **Geri:** Titrate dose carefully in elderly patients; **OB:** Use during pregnancy only if potential benefit justifies risk to the fetus; **Pedi:** Safety and effectiveness have not been established in children <17 yr.

Adverse Reactions/Side Effects
CNS: dizziness, headache, syncope, vertigo. **EENT:** diplopia. **CV:** PR interval prolongation. **GI:** nausea, vomiting. **Neuro:** ataxia. **Misc:** multiorgan hypersensitivity reactions (Drug Reaction with eosinophilia and systemic symptoms—DRESS).

Interactions
Drug-Drug: Use cautiously with other **drugs that affect cardiac conduction**.

Route/Dosage
PO, IV (Adults): 50 mg twice daily; may be increased weekly by 100 mg/day in two divided doses up to a maintenance dose of 200–400mg/day given in two divided doses *Severe renal impairment (CCR ≤30 ml/min) or mild to moderate hepatic impairment*— daily dose should not exceed 300 mg.

Availability
Tablets: 50 mg, 150 mg, 200 mg. **Solution for IV injection:** 200mg/20 mL single-use vials, 200 mg.

NURSING IMPLICATIONS

Assessment
- Assess location, duration, and characteristics of seizure activity. Institute seizure precautions.
- Monitor closely for notable changes in behavior that could indicate the

emergence or worsening of suicidal thoughts or behavior or depression.
- Assess ECG prior to therapy in patients with pre-existing cardiac disease.
- **Lab Test Considerations:** May cause ↑ ALT, which may return to normal without treatment.

Potential Nursing Diagnoses
Risk for injury (Indications)

Implementation
- IV administration is indicated for short term replacement when PO administration is not feasible. When switching from PO to IV, initial total daily dose should be equivalent to total daily dose and frequency of PO therapy. At end of IV period, may switch to PO at equivalent daily dose and frequency of IV therapy.
- **PO:** May be administered with or without food.

IV Administration
- **Intermittent Infusion: *Diluent:*** May be administered undiluted. ***Concentration:*** 10 mg/mL, or diluted with 0.9% NaCl, D5W, or LR.Solution is clear and colorless; do not administer solutions that are discolored or contain a precipitate. Solution is stable for 24 hr at room temperature. Discard unused portion. ***Rate:*** Infuse over 30–60 min.

Patient/Family Teaching
- Instruct patient to take lacosamide around the clock, as directed. Medication should be gradually discontinued over at least 1 wk to prevent seizures. Advise patient to read the *Medication Guide* before starting therapy and with each Rx refill.
- May cause dizziness, ataxia, and syncope. Caution patient to avoid driving or other activities requiring alertness until response to medication is known. Tell patient not to resume driving until physician gives clearance based on control of seizure disorder. If syncope occurs, advise patient to lay down with legs raised until recovered and notify health care professional.
- Inform patients and families of risk of suicidal thoughts and behavior and advise that behavioral changes, emergency or worsening signs and symptoms of depression, unusual changes in mood, or emergence of suicidal thoughts, behavior, or thoughts of self-harm should be reported to health care professional immediately.
- Instruct patient to notify health care professional if signs of multiorgan hypersensitivity reactions (fever, rash, fatigue, jaundice, dark urine) occur.
- Advise patient to consult health care professional before taking other Rx, OTC, or herbal preparation and to avoid taking alcohol or other CNS depressants concurrently with lacosamide.
- Advise female patients to notify health care professional if pregnancy is planned or suspected or if breast feeding. Encourage pregnant patients to enroll in the pregnancy registry by calling 1-888-537-7734.

Evaluation/Desired Outcomes
- Decreased seizure activity.

levoleucovorin calcium
(lee-vo-loo-koe-**vor**-in **kal**-see-um)
Fusilev

Classification
Thera: antidotes (for methotrexate), vitamins
Pharm: folic acid analogues

Pregnancy Category C

Indications

Used as "rescue" following high-dose methotrexate treatment of osteosarcoma. Decreases toxicity which may follow impaired methotrexate elimination or unintended toxicity of other folic acid antagonists.

Action

The reduced form of folic acid that serves as a cofactor in the synthesis of DNA and RNA; does not require dihydrofolate reductase for activity. **Therapeutic Effects:** Reversal of toxic effects of folic acid antagonists, including methotrexate, that inhibit dihydrofolate reductase.

Pharmacokinetics

Absorption: IV administration results on complete bioavailability.
Distribution: Transported actively and passively across cell membranes; enters CSF.
Metabolism and Excretion: Extensively converted to tetrahydrofolic derivatives.
Half-life: *Total tetrahydrofolic acid*—5.1 hr.

TIME/ACTION PROFILE

ROUTE	ONSET	PEAK	DURATION
IV	unknown	end of infusion	3–6 hr

Contraindications/Precautions

Contraindicated in: Hypersensitivity to folic acid or folinic acid.
Use Cautiously in: Concurrent use of anticonvulsants; may increase risk of seizures; **OB:** Use in pregnancy only if clearly needed, use cautiously during lactation; **Pedi:** Has been used safely in pediatric patients.

Adverse Reactions/Side Effects

(all patients also received methotrexate). **CNS:** confusion. **Resp:** dyspnea. **GI:** nausea, stomatitis, vomiting, altered taste, diarrhea, dyspepsia. **Derm:** dermatitis. **GU:** abnormal renal function. **Neuro:** neuropathy. **Misc:** allergic reactions.

Interactions

Drug-Drug: ↑ risk of toxicity from **fluorouracil**. May ↓ effectiveness of **phenobarbital**, **phenytoin**, or **primidone** leading to ↑ risk of seizures. May ↓ effectiveness of **trimethoprim-sulfamethoxazole** when used to treat *Pneumocustis carnii* pneumonia in HIV-infected patients.

Route/Dosage

Levoleucovorin rescue following high dose methotrexate—based on a methotrexate dose of 12 grams/m² IV over 4 hr and concurrent with hydration and maintenance of urine pH ≥7.0.

IV (Adults): *Normal methotrexate elimination*—7.5 mg (5 mg/m²) every 6 hr for 10 doses starting 24 hr after the start of the methotrexate infusion; *Delayed late methotrexate elimination*—7.5 mg (5 mg/m²) every 6 hr starting 24 hr after the start of the methotrexate infusion; continue until methotrexate level <5 × 10⁻⁸ (0.05 micromolar); *delayed early methotrexate elimination and/or evidence of acute renal injury*—75 mg (5 mg/m²) every 3 hr starting 24 hr after the start of the methotrexate infusion; continue until methotrexate level is <1 micromolar, then 7.5 mg every 3 hr until 0.05 micromolar).

Levoleucovorin rescue following inadvertent overdosage of methotrexate.

IV (Adults): 7.5 mg (approximately 5 mg/m²) every 6 hr until serum methotrexate level is less than 10⁻⁸ M. Determine creatinine and methotrexate levels at 24 hr intervals. If 24 hour serum creatinine has increased 50% over baseline or 24 hr methotrexate level is greater than 5×10^{-6} M or 48 hr level is greater than 9×10^{-7} M, ↑ dose to 50 mg/m² IV every 3 hr until methotrexate level is less than 10^{-8} M. Maintain hydration and urinary alkalinization (pH ≥7.0). Initiate as soon as possible and within 24 hr of methotrexate when there is delayed excretion; as time interval increases, effectiveness ↓ .

Availability
Lyophylized powder for injection (requires reconstitution: 50 mg vial (contains mannitol).

NURSING IMPLICATIONS

Assessment
- Assess patient for nausea and vomiting secondary to methotrexate therapy or folic acid antagonists (pyrimethamine and trimethoprim) overdose.
- Monitor for development of allergic reactions (rash, urticaria, wheezing). Notify physician if these occur.
- *Lab Test Considerations:* Monitor serum methotrexate and creatinine at least once daily levels to determine dosage and effectiveness of therapy. Leucovorin calcium levels should be equal to or greater than methotrexate level. Rescue continues until serum methotrexate level is $<5 \times 10^{-8}$ M.
- Monitor electrolytes and hydration status, and urine pH every 6 hr during therapy; pH should be maintained >7 to decrease nephrotoxic effects of high-dose methotrexate.

Potential Nursing Diagnoses
Risk for injury (Indications)
Imbalanced nutrition: less than body requirements (Indications)

Implementation
- **General:** Levoleucovorin is dosed at one-half the usual dose of the racemic form.

IV Administration
- **Intermittent Infusion:** Reconstitute 50 mg vial with 5.3 mL of 0.9% NaCl without preservatives for a concentration of 10 mg/mL. *Diluent:* Dilute further immediately in 0.9% NaCl or D5W. *Concentration:* 0.5 mg/mL–5 mg/mL. Initial reconstitution or dilutions in 0.9% NaCl are stable at room temperature for 12 hr. Dilutions in D5W are stable for 4 hrs at room temperature. Do not administer solutions that are cloudy or contain a precipitate. *Rate:* Administer at no more than 16 mL of reconstituted solution (160 mg levoleucovorin) per min; due to calcium content of solution.
- **Additive Incompatibility:** Do not admix with other solutions.

Patient/Family Teaching
- Explain purpose of medication to patient.

Evaluation/Desired Outcomes
- Reversal of toxic effects of methotrexate or in overdose of folic acid antagonists.

---

methoxypolyethylene glycol-epoetin beta
(meh-**thok**-see-**pah**-lee-**eh**-thih-leen **gly**-kol ee-**poh**-eh-tin **bay**-ta)
Mircera

Classification
Thera: antianemics
Pharm: hormones

Pregnancy Category C

Indications
Anemia due to chronic renal failure.

Action
Stimulates erythropoesis (production of red blood cells). **Therapeutic Ef-**

fects: Maintains and may elevate RBCs, decreasing the need for transfusions.

Pharmacokinetics

Absorption: Well absorbed (62%) following subcutaneous administration; IV administration results in complete bioavailability.
Distribution: Unknown.
Metabolism and Excretion: Unknown.
Half-life: 134 hr.

TIME/ACTION PROFILE (effect on hemoglobin)

ROUTE	ONSET	PEAK	DURATION
IV, Subcut	7–15 days	unknown	2–4 wk

Contraindications/Precautions

Contraindicated in: Hypersensitivity; Uncontrolled hypertension; Treatment of anemia due to cancer chemotherapy.
Use Cautiously in: Patients with hypertension or cardiovascular disease (monitor closely); Dialysis patients (IV route recommended to decrease immunogenecity); Predialysis patients (may require lower doses); **Geri:** Use lower doses, consider age related decrease in metabolic function, concurrent disease states and medications; **OB, Lactation:** Use during pregnancy only if maternal benefit outweighs fetal risk; **Pedi:** Safe use not established.

Adverse Reactions/Side Effects

CNS: SEIZURES, headaches. **CV:** CARDIOVASCULAR AND THROMBOTIC EVENTS, hypertension, hypotension. **GI:** diarrhea, constipation, vomiting. **Hemat:** PURE RED APLASIA. **Misc:** allergic reactions including ANAPHYLAXIS, fistula complications.

Interactions

Drug-Drug: None noted.

Route/Dosage

Subcut, IV (Adults): 0.6 mcg/kg once every two wk, dosing based on hemoglobin values. Once every-two-wk dose is determined, may be given monthly at twice the every-two-wk dose.

Availability

Vials of solution for injection: 50 mcg/mL, 100 mcg/mL, 200 mcg/mL, 300 mcg/mL, 400 mcg/mL, 600 mcg/mL, 1000 mcg/mL. **Prefilled syringes of solution:** 50 mcg/0.3 mL, 75 mcg/0.3 mL, 100 mcg/0.3 mL, 150 mcg/0.3 mL, 200 mcg/0.3 mL, 250 mcg/0.3 mL, 400 mcg/0.6 mL, 600 mcg/0.6 mL, 800 mcg/0.6 mL.

NURSING IMPLICATIONS

Assessment

- Monitor blood pressure closely before and during therapy, especially in patients with history of CV disease or hypertension. If blood pressure cannot be controlled, dose should be reduced or medication held.
- Monitor for signs of allergic reactions (tachycardia, pruritis, rash, wheezing, dyspnea, dizziness, fainting, swelling of around mouth or eyes, sweating). If signs occur, discontinue therapy and provide supportive care.
- May cause seizure. Assess neurological status periodically during therapy, especially if hemoglobin increases > 1 g/dL in any 2–wk period.
- Monitor response for symptoms of anemia (fatigue, dyspnea, pallor).
- *Lab Test Considerations:* Monitor hematocrit before and every 2 wks during initial therapy or dose adjustments until stabilized, and every 2–4 wks thereafter. Maintain hemoglobin between 10–12 g/dL. Do not adjust dose more often than once monthly; may require up to 6

wks for significant changes to occur. To adjust dose, increase or decrease by 25% as needed. During therapy, if hemoglobin approaches 12 g/dL or increases by >1 g/dL in any 2–wk period, reduce dose by 25%. If hemoglobin continues to increase, discontinue medication until hemoglobin begins to decrease, then restart at a dose 25% lower than previous dose. For patients not converted from another erythropoesis-stimulating agents (ESA), if the hemoglobin increase is <1 g/dL over the initial 4 wks and iron stores are adequate, may increase dose by 25%. If hemoglobin dose not reach 10–12 g/dL despite dose titration over 12 wks, do not administer higher doses and use lowest dose that will maintain hemoglobin sufficient to avoid recurrent RBC transfusions, evaluate and treat for other causes of anemia (deficiencies of iron, folic acid, vitamin B_{12}, and discontinue methoxy polyethylene glycol-epoetin beta if responsiveness does not improve and recurrent RBC transfusions are needed.

- May cause pure red cell aplasia (PRCA) and anemia. If a sudden loss of response to medication accompanied by severe anemia and low reticulocyte counts occur evaluate for development of neutralizing antibodies to erythropoetin. Obtain serum samples at least 1 mo after last dose to prevent interference with assay. If anti-erythropoetin antibody-associated anemia is suspected, withhold ESAs until confirmed. If confirmed, discontinue permanently all ESAs.
- Serum ferritin, transferrin, and iron levels should also be monitored to assess need for concurrent iron therapy. Transferrin saturation

should be at least 20% and ferritin should be at least 100 mcg/mL.
- Monitor renal function studies and electrolytes closely.

Potential Nursing Diagnoses
Activity intolerance (Indications)
Noncompliance (Patient/Family Teaching)

Implementation
- When converting patients from other ESAs dose can be administered once every 2 wks or once monthly based on the total weekly at the time of conversion. Patients receiving epoetin <8000 units or darbopoietin <40 mcg in the previous week should receive 120 mcg/month or 60 mcg of *Mircera* every 2 wks. Patients receiving epoetin 8000–16000 units or darbopoetin 40–80 mcg in the previous week should receive 200 mcg/month or 100 mcg *Mircera* every 2 wks. Patients receiving epoetin >16000 units or darbopoetin >80 mcg in the previous week should receive 360 mcg/month or 180 mcg *Mircera* every 2 wks.
- Patients not requiring dialysis may require lower maintenance doses.
- If a dose is missed, administer missed dose as soon as possible and restart at the previous dosing frequency.
- Transfusions are still required for severe symptomatic anemia. Supplemental iron should be continued throughout therapy.
- Avoid shaking or prolonged exposure to light; inactivation of medication may occur. Store in refrigerator; do not freeze. Vials are stable for up to 7 days and prefilled syringes for up to 30 days at room temperature. Discard vial or syringe immediately after withdrawing dose. Discard unused portions; do not pool or reuse.

Solution is colorless to slightly yellow; do not administer solutions that are discolored or contain particulate matter.

- **Subcut:** May be administered in outer area of upper arms, front of middle thighs, or abdomen, except for two-inch area around navel. Do not inject in areas that are tender, red, bruised, hard, or that has scars or stretch marks. Pinch skin and inject at a 45° or 90° angle.
- For administration using prefilled syringe, plunger must be fully depressed and full dose given during injection in order for the needle guard to activate. Following administration, remove needle from injection site and release plunger to allow the needle guard to move up until entire needle is covered.
- **Direct IV:** Administer undiluted. *Rate:* May be administered as direct injection or bolus into venous port of dialysis tubing at end of dialysis session.
- **Additive Incompatibility:** Do not mix with any parenteral solution.

Patient/Family Teaching

- Explain rationale for concurrent iron therapy (increased red blood cell production requires iron).
- Discuss ways of preventing self-injury in patients at risk for seizures. Driving and activities requiring continuous alertness should be avoided.
- Stress importance of compliance with dietary restrictions, medications, and dialysis. Foods high in iron and low in potassium include liver, pork, veal, beef, mustard and turnip greens, peas, eggs, broccoli, kale, blackberries, strawberries, apple juice, watermelon, oatmeal, and enriched bread. Medication will result in increased sense of well-being, but it does not cure underlying disease.
- Instruct patient to consult health care professional before taking any Rx, OTC, or vitamins, herbal products during therapy.
- Advise patient to notify health care professional immediately if chest pain; difficulty breathing or shortness of breath; pain in legs with or without swelling; a cool or pale arm or leg; sudden confusion or trouble speaking or understanding speech; sudden numbness or weakness of face, arm, or leg, especially in one side of body; sudden trouble seeing in one or both eyes; sudden trouble walking, dizziness, loss of balance or coordination, loss of consciousness; sudden severe headache with no known cause; seizures; or blood clots in hemodialysis vascular access occur.
- Advise female patient to notify health care professional if pregnancy is planned or suspected or if breastfeeding.
- Emphasize the need for regular blood pressure monitoring and lab tests for hemoglobin to decrease risks of serious of serious CV adverse effects.
- **Home Care Issues:** Home dialysis patients determined to be able to safely and effectively administer medication and should be taught proper dose, administration technique, and disposal of equipment. Inform patient that injection site reactions (redness, swelling, itching) may occur. Advise patient to rotate injection sites and to notify health care professional if a lump, swelling, or bruising at the injection site occurs and does not go away. *Medication Guide and Patient Instructions for Use* should be provided to

patient along with medication. Caution patient not to give medication to others, even if they have the same symptoms; may cause harm.

Evaluation/Desired Outcomes
• Increase in hemoglobin and maintenance of 10–12 g/dL with improvement in symptoms of anemia in patients with chronic renal failure.

---

methylnatrexone
(me-thil-nal-**trex**-one)
Relistor
Classification
Thera: laxatives
Pharm: opioid antagonists

Pregnancy Category B

Indications
Treatment of constipation caused by opioid use in patients being treated palliatively, when laxative therapy has failed.

Action
Acts peripherally as mu-opioid receptor antagonist, blocking opioid effects on the GI tract. **Therapeutic Effects:** Blocks constipating effects of opioids on the GI tract without loss of analgesia.

Pharmacokinetics
Absorption: Absorption follows subcutaneous administration.
Distribution: Moderate tissue distribution, does not cross the blood-brain barrier.
Metabolism and Excretion: Some metabolism, 85% excreted unchanged in urine.
Half-life: 8 hr.

TIME/ACTION PROFILE

ROUTE	ONSET	PEAK	DURATION
Subcut	rapid	0.5 hr	24–48 hr

Contraindications/Precautions
Contraindicated in: Known/suspected mechanical GI obstruction.
Use Cautiously in: OB, Lactation: Use in pregnancy only if clearly needed; use cautiously during lactation; **Pedi:** Safety and efficacy in children not established.

Adverse Reactions/Side Effects
CNS: dizziness. **GI:** <u>abdominal pain</u>, diarrhea, <u>flatulence</u>, <u>nausea</u>.

Interactions
Drug-Drug: None noted.

Route/Dosage
Subcut: (Adults): *38– <62 kg*—8 mg every other day, not to exceed every 24 hr; *62–114 kg*—12 mg every other day, not to exceed every 24 hr; *other weights* 0.15 mg/kg every other day, not to exceed every 24 hr
Renal Impairment
(Adults): *CCr <30 ml/min*—use 50% of recommended dose based on weight.

Availability
Solution for subcutaneous injection: 12mg/0.6 mL single use vial.

NURSING IMPLICATIONS

Assessment
• Assess bowel sounds and frequency, quantity, and consistency of stools periodically during therapy.
• Monitor pain intensity during therapy. Methylnaltrexone does not affect pain or effects of opioid analgesics on pain control.

Potential Nursing Diagnoses
Constipation (Indications)
Diarrhea (Adverse Reactions)

Implementation
• **Subcut:** Pinch skin and administer in upper arm, abdomen, or thigh at a 45° angle using a 1 mL syring with a 27-gauge needle inserted the full

---

length of the needle. Do not rub the injection site. Solution is clear and colorless to pale yellow. Do not administer solutions that are discolored or contain a precipitate. Solution is stable for 24 hr at room temperature. Protect vials from light. Do not freeze. Do not use single-use vials for more than 1 dose.

Patient/Family Teaching

- Instruct patient on administration of methylnaltrexone and disposal of supplies. Usual schedule is one dose every other day, as needed, but no more than one dose in a 24 hr period. Advise patient to read the *Patient Information* prior to starting therapy and with each Rx refill.
- Advise patient that laxation may occur within 30 min, so toilet facilities should be available following administration.
- May cause dizziness. Caution patient to avoid driving and other activities requiring alertness until response to medication is known.
- Advise patient to notify health care professional and discontinue therapy if severe or persistent diarrhea occurs or if abdominal pain, nausea, or vomiting persists or worsens.
- Instruct patient to stop taking methylnaltrexone if they stop taking opioid medications.
- Advise patient to consult health care professional prior to taking other Rx, OTC, or herbal products.
- Advise female patients to notify health care professional if pregnancy is planned or suspected or if breastfeeding.

Evaluation/Desired Outcomes

- Laxation and relief of opioid-induced constipation.

milnacipran
(mil-na-**sip**-ran)
Savella

Classification
Thera: antifibromyalgia agents
Pharm: selective norepinephrine reuptake inhibitors

Pregnancy Category C

Indications
Management of fibromyalgia.

Action
Inhibits neuronal reuptake of norepinephrine and serotonin. **Therapeutic Effects:** Decreased pain associated with fibromyalgia.

Pharmacokinetics
Absorption: 85–90% absorbed following oral administration.
Distribution: Unknown.
Metabolism and Excretion: Mostly excreted urine as unchanged drug (55%) and inactive metabolites.
Half-life: *D*-isomer 8–10 hr; *L*-isomer 4–6 hr.

TIME/ACTION PROFILE (decrease in pain)

ROUTE	ONSET	PEAK	DURATION
PO	1 wk	unknown	unknown

Contraindications/Precautions
Contraindicated in: Uncontrolled narrow-angle glaucoma; Concurrent use of or in close temporal proximity to MAO inhibitors; End-stage renal disease; Significant history of alcohol use/abuse; Chronic liver disease.
Use Cautiously in: History of suicide risk or attempt; History of seizures; Moderate-to-severe renal impairment; for CCr <30 mL/min reduced dose is required; Severe hepatic impairment; Obstructive uropathy (↑ risk of ad-

verse genitourinary effects); **Geri:** Consider age-related decrease in renal function, chronic disease state and concurrent drug therapy; **OB:** Use only if clearly required during pregnancy weighing benefit to mother versus potential harm to fetus; **Lactation:** Potential for serious adverse reactions in infant; discontinue drug or discontinue breastfeeding; **Pedi:** Increased risk of suicidal thinking and behavior (suicidality) in adolescents and young adults up to 24 yrs with Major Depressive Disorder (MDD) and other psychiatric disorders.

Adverse Reactions/Side Effects

CNS: dizziness, headache, insomnia. **CV:** hypertension, tachycardia. **GI:** constipation, dry mouth, liver function abnormalities, nausea, vomiting. **Derm:** hot flushes, hyperhydrosis.

Interactions

Drug-Drug: Concurrent use with **MAO inhibitors** may result in serious, potentially fatal reactions; wait at least 14 days following discontinuation of MAO inhibitor before initiation of milnacipran Wait at least 5 days after discontinuing. milnacipran before initiation of MAO inhibitor. Concurrent use with **MAO inhibitors** may result in serious, potentially fatal reactions; wait at least 14 days following discontinuation of MAO inhibitor before initiation of milnacipran Wait at least 5 days after discontinuing. milnacipran before initiation of MAO inhibitor. Concurrent use of **serotonergic drugs** (including **triptans**, **lithium**, and **tramadol**) may ↑ the risk of serotinin syndrome; also ↑ risk of coronary vasoconstriction and hypertension. Concurrent use of **NSAIDs**, **aspirin**, or other **drugs that affect coagulation** may ↑ the risk of bleeding. May ↓ antihypertensive effectiveness of **clonidine**. ↑ risk of hypertension and arrhythmias with

epinephrine or **norepinephrine**. ↑ risk of euphoria and hypotension when switching from **clomipramine**. Concurrent use with **digoxin** may result in adverse hemodynamics, including hypotension and tachycardia; avoid concurrent use with IV digoxin.

Route/Dosage

PO (Adults): *Day 1*—12.5 mg; *Day 2–3*— 12.5 mg twice daily; *Day 4–7*— 25 mg twice daily; *After Day 7*— 50 mg twice daily. Some patients may be require up to 100 mg twice daily depending on response.

Renal Impairment

PO (Adults): *CCr 5–29 mL/min*— maintenance dose is 25 mg twice daily; some patients may be require up to 50 mg twice daily depending on response.

Availability

Tablets (contain tartrazine): 12.5 mg, 25 mg, 50 mg, 100 mg.

NURSING IMPLICATIONS

Assessment

- Assess intensity, quality, and location of pain periodically during therapy. May require several wk for effects to be seen.
- Monitor blood pressure and heart rate before and periodically during therapy. Treat per-existing hypertension and cardiac disease prior to therapy. Sustained hypertension may be dose related; decrease dose or discontinue therapy if this occurs.
- Monitor closely for notable changes in behavior that could indicate the emergence or worsening of suicidal thoughts or behavior or depression.
- *Lab Test Considerations:* May cause ↑ ALT, AST, and bilirubin.

Potential Nursing Diagnoses

Chronic pain (Indications)
Risk for suicide (Adverse Reactions)

Implementation

- **PO:** May be administered without regard to meals; may be more tolerable if taken with food.

Patient/Family Teaching

- Instruct patient to take milnacipran as directed at the same time each day. Take missed doses as soon as possible unless time for next dose. Do not stop abruptly; must be decreased gradually. Advise patient to read the *Medication Guide* prior to therapy and with each Rx refill.
- Encourage patient and family to be alert for emergence of anxiety, agitation, panic attacks, insomnia, irritability, hostility, impulsivity, akathisia, hypomania, mania, worsening of depression and suicidal ideation, especially during early antidepressant therapy. Assess symptoms on a day-to-day basis as changes may be abrupt. If these symptoms occur, notify health care professional.
- May cause dizziness. Caution patient to avoid driving or other activities requiring alertness until response to medication is known.
- Advise patient to consult health care professional prior to taking any Rx, OTC, or herbal products. Avoid use of aspirin, NSAIDs, and warfarin due to increased risk for bleeding.
- Instruct patient to notify health care professional if signs of liver damage (pruritus, dark urine, jaundice, right upper quadrant tenderness, unexplained "flu-like" symptoms) or hyponatremia (headache, difficulty concentrating, memory impairment, confusion, weakness, unsteadiness) occur.
- Advise patient to avoid taking alcohol during milnacipran therapy.
- Instruct patient to notify health care professional if pregnancy is planned or suspected or if breastfeeding.

- Encourage patient to maintain routine follow-up visits with health care provider to determine effectiveness.

Evaluation/Desired Outcomes

- Reduction in pain and soreness associated with fibromyalgia.

---

nebivolol (ne-**bi**-vi-lole)
Bystolic
Classification
Thera: antihypertensives
Pharm: beta blockers (selective)

Pregnancy Category C

Indications

Hypertension (alone and with other antihypertensives).

Action

Blocks stimulation of beta adrenergic receptor sites; selective for beta₁ (myocardial) receptors in most patients. In some patients (poor metabolizers, higher blood levels may result in some beta₂ [pulmonary, vascular, uterine] adrenergic) blockade. **Therapeutic Effects:** Lowering of blood pressure.

Pharmacokinetics

Absorption: Well absorbed following oral administration.
Distribution: Unknown.
Protein Binding: 98%.
Metabolism and Excretion: Mostly metabolized by the liver, including the CYP2D6 enzyme system; some have antihypertensive action; minimal excretion of unchanged drug.
Half-life: *Extensive metabolizers—* 12 hr; *poor metabolizers—*19 hr.

TIME/ACTION PROFILE (blood levels)

ROUTE	ONSET	PEAK	DURATION
PO	unknown	1.5–4 hr	24 hr

Contraindications/Precautions
Contraindicated in: Hypersensitivity; Severe bradycardia, heart block greater than first degree. cardiogenic shock, decompensated heart failure or sick sinus syndrome (without pacemaker); Severe hepatic impairment (Child-Pugh >B); Bronchospastic disease; **OB:** Lactation.

Use Cautiously in: Coronary artery disease (rapid cessation should be avoided); Compensated congestive heart failure; Major surgery (anesthesia may augment myocardial depression); Diabetes mellitus (may mask signs of hypoglycemia); Thyrotoxicosis (may mask symptoms); Moderate hepatic impairment (↓ metabolism); Severe renal impairment (↓ initial dose if CCr <30 ml/min); History of severe allergic reactions (↑ intensity of reactions); Pheochromocytoma (alpha blockers required prior to beta blockers); **Geri:** Consider increased sensitivity, concurrent chronic diseases, medications and presence of age-related decrease in clearance; **OB:** Use in pregnancy only if maternal benefit outweighs fetal risk; **Pedi:** Safe use in children <18 yr not established.

Adverse Reactions/Side Effects
CNS: dizziness, fatigue, headache.

Interactions
Drug-Drug: Drugs that affect the CYP2D6 enzyme system are expected to alter levels and possibly effects of nebivolol; dose alterations may be required. **Fluoxetine**, a known inhibitor of CYP2D6, ↑ levels and effects; similar effects may be expected from **quinidine**, **propafenone**, and **paroxetine**. Blood levels are also ↑ by **cimetine**. **Anesthetic agents** including **ether**, **trichloroethylene**, and **cyclopropane** as well as **other myocardial depressants** or **inhibitors of AV conduction** such as **diltiazem** and **verapamil** may ↑ risk of myocardial depression and bradycardia. Avoid concurrent use with **beta blockers**. Concurrent use with **reserpine** or **guanethidine** may excessively reduce sympathetic activity. If used concurrently with **clonidine**, nebivolol should be tapered and discontinued several days prior to gradual withdrawal of clonidine.

Route/Dosage
PO (Adults): 5 mg once daily initially, may increase at 2 wk intervals up to 40 mg/day.

Hepatic/Renal Impairment
PO (Adults): 2.5 mg once daily initially; titrate upward cautiously.

Availability
Tablets: 2.5, 5 mg, 10 mg.

NURSING IMPLICATIONS

Assessment
- Monitor blood pressure, ECG, and pulse prior to and periodically during therapy.
- Monitor intake and output ratios and daily weights. Assess routinely for signs and symptoms of CHF (dyspnea, rales/crackles, weight gain, peripheral edema, jugular venous distention).
- *Lab Test Considerations:* May cause ↑ BUN, uric acid, triglycerides and ↓ HDL cholesterol and platelet court.

Potential Nursing Diagnoses
Decreased cardiac output (Side Effects)

Implementation
- **PO:** May be administered without regard to food.
- When discontinuation is planned, observe patient carefully and advise to minimize physical activity. Taper over 1–2 wks when possible. If angina worsens or acute coronary insuf-

ficiency develops, reinstitute nebivolol promptly, at least temporarily.

Patient/Family Teaching

- Instruct patient to take nebivolol as
directed, at the same time each day,
even if feeling well. If a dose is
missed, skip missed dose and take
next scheduled dose; do not double
doses. Do not discontinue without
consulting health care professional.
Abrupt withdrawal may precipitate
life-threatening arrhythmias, hypertension, or myocardial ischemia.
- Advise patient to ensure that enough
medication is available for week-
ends, holidays, and vacations. A writ-
ten prescription may be kept in the
wallet for emergencies.
- Reinforce the need to continue additional therapies for hypertension
(weight loss, sodium restriction,
stress reduction, regular exercise,
moderation of alcohol consumption,
and smoking cessation). Medication
controls but does not cure
hypertension.
- Teach patient and family how to
check pulse and blood pressure. Instruct them to check pulse daily and
blood pressure biweekly and to report significant changes to health
care professional.
- Instruct patient to consult health
care professional before taking any
Rx, OTC, or herbal products, especially cold preparations, concurrently with this medication. Patients
on antihypertensive therapy should
also avoid excessive amounts of cof-
fee, tea, and cola.
- May mask some signs of hypoglycemia, especially tachycardia. Diabet-
ics should closely monitor blood
sugar, especially if weakness, mal-
aise, irritability, or fatigue occurs.
Medication does not block dizziness

or sweating as signs of
hypoglycemia.
- May cause dizziness. Caution patients to avoid driving or other activities requiring alertness until response to medication is known.
- Advise patient to notify health care
professional if difficulty breathing or
signs and symptoms of worsening
CHF (weight gain, increasing
shortness or breath, excessive
bradycardia) occur.
- Instruct patient to inform health care
professional of medication regimen
before treatment or surgery.
- Advise patient to carry identification
describing disease process and
medication regimen at all times.
- Advise female patients that breastfeeding should be avoided during
nebivolol therapy.

Evaluation/Desired Outcomes

- Decrease in blood pressure.

nilotinib (ni-lo-ti-nib)
Tasigna
Classification
Thera: antineoplastics
Pharm: enzyme inhibitors, ki-
nase inhibitors

Pregnancy Category D

Indications

Chronic or accelerated phase Philadel-
phia chromosome positive chronic my-
elogenous leukemia which has not responded to other treatment, including
imatinib.

Action

Inhibits kinases which may be pro-
duced by malignant cell lines. **Therapeutic Effects:** Inhibits production of
malignant cells lines with decreased
proliferation of leukemic cells.

Pharmacokinetics

Absorption: Well absorbed following oral administration. Blood levels are significantly increased by food.

Distribution: Unknown.

Metabolism and Excretion: Mostly metabolized by the liver; metabolites are not active.

Half-life: 17 hr.

TIME/ACTION PROFILE (blood levels)

ROUTE	ONSET	PEAK	DURATION
PO	unknown	3 hr	12 hr

Contraindications/Precautions

Contraindicated in: Hypokalemia or hypomagnesemia; Long QT syndrome; Concurrent use of medications known to prolong QT interval; Concurrent use of strong inhibitors of the CYP3A4 enzyme system (increased risk of toxicity); Concurrent use of strong inducers of the CYP3A4 enzyme system (may ↓ effectiveness); Concurrent grapefruit juice (may ↑ risk of toxicity); Galactose intolerance, severe lactase deficiency or glucose-galactose malabsorption (capsules contain lactose); **OB:** Pregnancy or lactation.

Use Cautiously in: Concurrent use of other drugs that prolong QT interval; Electrolyte abnormalities; correct prior to administration to ↓ risk of arrhythmias; Hepatic impairment (↓ dose required for Grade 3 elevated bilirubin, transaminases or lipase); **OB:** Women with child-bearing potential (effective contraception required); **Pedi:** Safe use in children has not been established.

Adverse Reactions/Side Effects

CNS: <u>fatigue</u>, <u>headache</u>, dizziness. **EENT:** vertigo. **CV:** ARRHYTHMIAS, hypertension, palpitations, QT prolongation. **GI:** <u>constipation</u>, <u>diarrhea</u>, <u>nausea</u>, <u>vomiting</u>, abdominal discomfort, anorexia, dyspepsia, flatulence, hepatotoxicity. **Derm:** <u>pruritus</u>, <u>rash</u>, alopecia, flushing. **F and E:** hyperkalemia, hypocalcemia, hypokalemia, hyponatremia, hypophosphatemia. **Hemat:** <u>MYELOSUPRESSION</u>. **Metab:** ↑ lipase, hyperglycemia. **MS:** musculoskeletal pain. **Neuro:** paresthesia. **Misc:** <u>fever</u>, night sweats.

Interactions

Drug-Drug: Strong **inhibitors of the CYP3A4 enzyme system** including **ketoconazole**, **itraconaole**, **voriconazole**, **clarithromycin**, **telithromycin**, **atazanavir**, **indinavir**, **nelfinavir**, **indinavir**, **ritonavir**, **saquinavir**, and **nefazodone** may result in ↑ blood levels and toxicity and should be avoided; if concurrent use in necessary, dose reduction by 50% (400 mg once daily) may be required. Strong **inducers of the CYP3A4 enzyme system** including **carbamazepine**, **dexamethasone**, **phenobarbital**, **phenytoin**, **rifabutin**, **rifampin**, and **rifapentin** may ↓ blood levels and effectiveness and should be avoided if possible; if required, dose ↑ may be necessary. Nilotinib inhibits the following enzyme systems: **CYP3A4**, **CYP2C8**, **CYP2C9**, and **CYP2D6**; concurrent use of drugs metabolized by these systems may result in toxicity of these agents. Nilotinib induces the following enzyme systems: **CYP2D6**, **CYP2C8**, **CYP2C9**; concurrent use of drugs metabolized by these systems may result ↓ therapeutic effectiveness of these agents. Concurrent use of other **drugs that prolong QT interval**; may ↑ risk of serious arrhythmias.

Drug-Natural Products: *St. John's wort* may ↓ levels and effectiveness; avoid concurrent use.

Drug-Food: **Grapefruit juice** may ↑ blood levels and should be avoided.

Route/Dosage
PO (Adults): 400 mg twice daily; adjustment may be required for toxicity and/or drug interactions.

Availability
Capsules: 200 mg.

NURSING IMPLICATIONS

Assessment
- Monitor ECG to assess the QTc interval at baseline, 7 days after initiation of therapy, and periodically thereafter. For ECGs with QTc >480 msec, withhold nilotinib and check serum potassium and magnesium. If below lower limit of normal, correct to normal with supplements. Review concommitant medications for effects on electrolytes. If QTc returns to <450 msec and within 20 msec of baseline within 2 wks, return ot prior dose. If QTc is <480 msec and >450 msec after 2 wks, reduce nilotinib dose to 400 mg once daily. Following dose reduction to 400 mg once daily, if QTc return to >480 msec, discontinue nilotinib. Repeat ECG approximately 7 days after any dose adjustment.
- Monitor for myelosuppression. Assess for bleeding (bleeding gums, bruising, petechiae, blood in stools, urine, emesis) and avoid IM injections and taking rectal temperatures if platelet count is low. Apply pressure to venipuncture sites for at least 10 min. Assess for signs of infection during neutropenia. Anemia may occur. Monitor for fatigue, dyspnea, and othrostatic hypotension.
- *Lab Test Considerations:* Monitor serum electrolytes prior to and periodically during therapy. May cause hypokalemia, hypomagnesemia, hypophosphatemia, hyperkalemia, hypocalcemia, hyperglycemia, and hyponatremia.

- Monitor CBC every 2 wks for first 2 mo and monthly thereafter or as indicated. May cause Grade 3/4 thrombocytopenia, neutropenia, and anemia. If ANC is $<1.0 \times 10^9$/L and/or platelet counts $<50 \times 10^9$/L, stop nilotinib and monitor blood counts. Resume within 2 wks at prior dose if ANC $>1.0 \times 10^9$/L and platelets $>50 \times 10^9$/L. If blood counts remain low for >2 wks, reduce dose to 400 mg once daily. Myelosuppression is generally reversible.
- May cause ↑ serum lipase or amylase. If ↑ to ≥Grade 3, withhold nilotinib and monitor serum levels. Resume treatment at 400 mg once daily if serum lipase or amylase return to ≤Grade 1.
- May cause ↑ serum bilirubin. If ↑ to ≥Grade 3, withhold nilotinib and monitor bilirubin. Resume treatment at 400 mg once daily if serum lipase or amylase return to ≤Grade 1.
- May cause ↑ serum hepatic tranaminases. If ↑ to ≥Grade 3, withhold nilotinib and monitor serum ALT, AST, and alkaline phosphatase. Resume treatment at 400 mg once daily if serum lipase or amylase return to ≤Grade 1.

Potential Nursing Diagnoses
Deficient knowledge, related to medication regimen (Patient/Family Teaching)

Implementation
- **General:** Correct hypokalemia and hypomagnesemia prior to beginning therapy.
- **PO:** Administer twice daily at 12-hr intervals on an empty stomach, at least 1 hr before and 2 hrs after food. Capsule should be swallowed whole with water; do not open capsule.

Patient/Family Teaching

- Advise patient to take nilotinib as directed, approximately 12 hr apart. If a dose is missed, skip dose and resume taking next prescribed dose. Advise patients to avoid grapefruit products during therapy. Nilotinib is a long-term treatment; do not stop medication or change dose without consulting health care professional.
- May cause dizziness. Caution patient to avoid driving or other activities requiring alertness until response to medication is known.
- Advise patient to consult health care professional before taking any Rx, OTC, herbal, or vitamin products, especially St. John's Wort, during therapy.
- Instruct patient to notify health care professional promptly if fever; chills; cough; hoarseness; sore throat; signs of infection; Lower back or side pain; painful or difficulty urination; bleeding gums; bruising; petechiae; blood in stools, urine, or emesis; increased fatigue; dyspnea; or orthostatic hypotension occurs. Caution patient to avoid crowds and persons with known infections. Instruct patients to use a soft toothbrush and electric razor and to avoid falls. Caution patient not to drink alcoholic beverages or take medication containing aspirin or NSAIDs; may precipitate bleeding.
- Instruct patient not to receive any vaccinations without advice of health care professional.
- Discuss the possibility of hair loss with patient. Explore methods of coping. Regrowth usually occurs 2–3 mo after discontinuation of therapy.
- Advise women of childbearing potential to use effective contraception during therapy.

Evaluation/Desired Outcomes

- Decrease in production of leukemic cells.

---

olopatadine (nasal spray)
(o-lo-**pa**-ta-deen)
Patanase

Classification
Thera: allergy, cold, and cough remedies
Pharm: antihistamines

Pregnancy Category C

Indications
Relief of symptoms of allergic rhinitis.

Action
Antagonizes the effects of histamine at histamine₁ receptor sites; does not bind to or inactivate histamine. **Therapeutic Effects:** Decreased symptoms of histamine excess including rhinorrhea, sneezing and nasal itching.

Pharmacokinetics
Absorption: 57% absorbed from nasal mucosa.
Distribution: Unknown.
Metabolism and Excretion: Minimal metabolism; 70% eliminated in urine mostly as unchanged drug; 17% fecal elimination.
Half-life: 8–12 hr.

TIME/ACTION PROFILE

ROUTE	ONSET	PEAK	DURATION
Nasal	rapid	unknown	12 hr

Contraindications/Precautions
Contraindicated in: None noted;.
Use Cautiously in: Nasal pathology other than allergic rhinitis; **Geri:** Dose cautiously in elderly patients; consider age-related decrease in organ function and concurrent medications; **Lactation: OB:** Use in pregnancy or lactation

only when maternal benefit outweighs fetal risk; **Pedi:** Safe use in children <12 yr not established.

Adverse Reactions/Side Effects
CNS: drowsiness, headache. **EENT:** epistaxis, nasal perforation, nasal ulcerations, pharyngolaryngeal pain, post-nasal drip. **GI:** bitter taste. **Resp:** cough.

Interactions
Drug-Drug: ↑ CNS depression may occur with **alcohol**; avoid concurrent use.

Route/Dosage
Intranasal (Adults and Children ≥ 12 yr): 2 sprays in each nostril twice daily.

Availability
Nasal spray: 665 mcg/100 microliter (0.6%) spray in 30.5–g bottle (provides 240 metered sprays).

NURSING IMPLICATIONS

Assessment
- Assess for symptoms of seasonal allergic rhinitis (sneezing, runny nose, nasal itching) prior to and during therapy.

Potential Nursing Diagnoses
Ineffective airway clearance (Indications)

Implementation
- Administer 2 sprays per nostril twice daily.

Patient/Family Teaching
- Instruct patient to prime nasal spray by releasing 5 sprays or spraying until a fine mist appears before initial use. If unit has not been used within 7 days, re-prime with 2 sprays.
- May cause drowsiness. Advise patient to avoid driving or other activities that require alertness until response to medication is known.
- Instruct patient to avoid concurrent use of alcohol or other CNS depressants.

Evaluation/Desired Outcomes
- Relief of symptoms of seasonal allergic rhinitis.

oxybutynin transdermal gel (ox-i-**byoo**-ti-nin)
Gelnique
Classification
Thera: urinary tract antispasmodics
Pharm: anticholinergics
Pregnancy Category B

Indications
Treatment of overactive bladder.

Action
Inhibits the action of acetylcholine at postganglionic receptors. Has direct spasmolytic action on smooth muscle, including smooth muscle lining the GU tract, without affecting vascular smooth muscle. **Therapeutic Effects:** Decreased symptoms of overactive bladder including urge urinary incontinence, urgency and frequency.

Pharmacokinetics
Absorption: Absorbed through intact skin via passive diffusion.
Distribution: Widely distributed in body tissues.
Metabolism and Excretion: Extensively metabolized by the liver and in the intestinal mucosa (CYP3A4); one metabolite is pharmacologically active; metabolites are renally excreted with negligible (<0.1%) excretion of unchanged drug.
Half-life: 64 hr (following transdermal application).

TIME/ACTION PROFILE

ROUTE	ONSET	PEAK	DURATION
TD	unknown	unknown	24 hr

Contraindications/Precautions

Contraindicated in: Hypersensitivity; Urinary retention; Gastric retention; Uncontrolled narrow angle glaucoma. **Use Cautiously in:** Hepatic or renal impairment; Myasthenia gravis; Clinically significant bladder outflow obstruction; Ulcerative colitis, intestinal atony, gastroesophageal reflux; **OB: Lactation:** Use in pregnancy when probable clinical benefits outweigh possible hazards. Use cautiously during lactation; **Pedi:** Use in children has not been established.

Adverse Reactions/Side Effects

CNS: dizziness, fatigue, headache. **GI:** dry mouth, constipation. **Derm:** application site reactions, pruritus.

Interactions

Drug-Drug: Concurrent use of other **anticholinergic medications** may ↑ the risk/severity of dry mouth, constipation, blurred vision, somnolence and other anticholinergic effects.

Route/Dosage

PO (Adults): Apply contents of one sachet (100 mg/g) once daily.

Availability

10 %Gel: 1 g unit dose (sachet) contains 100 mg/g.

NURSING IMPLICATIONS

Assessment

- Monitor voiding pattern and intake and output ratios, and assess abdomen for bladder distention prior to and periodically during therapy.

Potential Nursing Diagnoses

Impaired urinary elimination (Indications)

Risk for injury (Side Effects)

Implementation

- **Transdermal:** Apply clear, colorless gel once daily to intact skin on abdomen (avoid area around navel), upper arms/shoulders, or thighs until dry. Rotate sites; do not use same site on consecutive days.

Patient/Family Teaching

- Instruct patient on correct application of oxybutinin gel. Do not apply to recently shaved skin, skin with rashes, or areas treated with lotions, oils, or powders; may be used with sunscreen. Wash area with mild soap and water and dry completely before applying. Tear packet open just before use and squeeze entire contents into hand or directly on to application site. Amount of gel will be size of a nickel on the skin. Gently rub into skin until dry. Wash hands immediately following application. Avoid application near open fire or when smoking; medication is flammable. Do not shower, bathe, swim, exercise, or immerse the application site in water within 1 hr after application. Cover application site with clothing if close skin-to-skin contact at application site is anticipated. Advise patient to read *Information for the Patient* prior to beginning therapy and with each Rx refill in case of new information.
- May cause drowsiness or blurred vision. Advise patient to avoid driving and other activities requiring alertness until response to medication is known.
- Advise patient to avoid concurrent use of alcohol and other CNS depressants while taking this medication.
- Instruct patient that frequent rinsing of mouth, good oral hygiene, and sugarless gum or candy may decrease dry mouth. Health care professional

should be notified if mouth dryness persists >2 wk.

- Advise patient to notify health care professional if rash develops; oxybutinin transdermal gel may be discontinued.
- Inform patient that oxybutynin decreases the body's ability to perspire. Avoid strenuous activity in a warm environment because overheating may occur.
- Advise patient to notify health care professional if urinary retention occurs or if constipation persists. Discuss methods of preventing constipation, such as increasing dietary bulk, increasing fluid intake, and increasing mobility.
- Instruct patient to consult health care professional before taking other Rx, OTC, or herbal products.
- Advise female patients to notify health care professional if pregnancy is planned or suspected or if breastfeeding.

Evaluation/Desired Outcomes

- Relief of symptoms (frequency, urgency, nocturia, and incontinence) in patients with overactive bladder.

---

plerixafor (ple-**rix**-fore)
Mozobil

Classification
Thera: none assigned
Pharm: hematopoietic stem cell mobilizers

Pregnancy Category D

Indications

Mobilizes hematopoietic stem cells to peripheral blood for collection and use in autologous transplantation in patients with non-Hodgkin's lymphoma and multiple myeloma; used in combination with granulocyte-colony stimulation factor (G-CSF).

Action

Inhibits the CXCR-4 chemokine receptor, blocking it's binding ability. Inhibition decreases adherence of stem cells to bone marrow, freeing them up to mobilize to peripheral blood. **Therapeutic Effects:** Mobilization of stem cells to peripheral blood allowing collection.

Pharmacokinetics

Absorption: Well absorbed following subcut administration.
Distribution: Largely confined to extravascular fluid space.
Metabolism and Excretion: Not metabolized by the liver; 70% unchanged in urine.
Half-life: 5.3 hr.

TIME/ACTION PROFILE (mobilization of cells)

ROUTE	ONSET	PEAK	DURATION
Subcut	rapid	10–14 hr*	unknow

*With G-CSF pretreatment.

Contraindications/Precautions

Contraindicated in: Leukemia; OB, **Lactation:** Pregnancy, lactation.
Use Cautiously in: Renal impairment (dose reduction required if CCr ≤50 mL/min); **Geri:** Consider age-related decrease in renal function and greater sensitivity to drug effects; **OB:** Women with child-bearing potential; **Pedi:** Safety and effectiveness in children have not been established.

Adverse Reactions/Side Effects

CNS: dizziness, fatigue, headache, insomnia. **GI:** SPLENIC RUPTURE, diarrhea, nausea, vomiting, abdominal distention/pain, constipation, dry mouth, dyspepsia, flatulence. **Derm:** erythema, sweating. **Hemat:** leukemia/tumor cell mobilization, thrombocytopenia. **Local:** <u>injection site reactions</u>. **MS:** musculoskeletal pain. **Neuro:** oral hypoesthesia.

Interactions
Drug-Drug: None noted.

Route/Dosage
Subcut: (Adults): *Following pretreatment with G-CSF for 4 days—* 0.24 mg/kg once daily for up to 4 days (not to exceed 40 mg/day); use actual body weight to calculate dose **Renal Impairment**
Subcut: (Adults): *Following pretreatment with G-CSF for 4 days—* 0.16 mg/kg once daily for up to 4 days (not to exceed 27 mg/day).

Availability
Solution for subcutaneous injection: 20 mg/mL in 1.2 mL vials.

NURSING IMPLICATIONS

Assessment
- Assess for splenic enlargement and potential rupture (left upper abdominal pain and/or scapular or shoulder pain) periodically during therapy.
- *Lab Test Considerations:* Monitor WBC and platelets during therapy. May cause leukocytosis and thrombocytopenia.

Potential Nursing Diagnoses
Deficient knowledge, related to medication regimen (Patient/Family Teaching)

Implementation
- Begin therapy after patient has received 4 days of G-CSF daily and approximately 11 hrs prior to initiation of apheresis.
- **Subcut:** Administer subcut daily for 4 days. Do not use solutions that are discolored or contain a precipitate. Vials are single use; discard any unused medication.

Patient/Family Teaching
- Explain purpose of medication to patient.
- Advise patient to report signs and symptoms of potential systemic reactions (urticaria, periorbital swelling, dyspnea, hypoxia) to health care professional.
- Instruct patient to notify health care professional immediately if vasovagal reactions (orthostatic hypotension, syncope) occur during or shortly after injection.
- Advise patient to notify health care professional if itching, rash, or reactions at injection site occur; may be treated with OTC medications.
- May cause GI disorders including diarrhea, nausea, vomiting, flatulence, and abdominal pain. Advise patient to notify health care professional if GI disorders are severe.
- Plerixafor is teratogenic. Caution female patients to use effective contraception during therapy and to notify health care professional if pregnancy is planned or suspected or if breastfeeding.

Evaluation/Desired Outcomes
- Increase in CD34+ cells/kg in peripheral blood prior to aphresis.

---

raltegravir (ral-**teg**-ra-veer)
Isentress
Classification
Thera: antiretrovirals
Pharm: integrase strand transfer inhibitor (INSTI)

Pregnancy Category C

Indications
HIV infection (with other antiretrovirals) in patients who are failing other treatments as evidenced by continued

viral replication and resistance to other agents.

Action
Inhibits HIV-1 integrase, which is required for viral replication. **Therapeutic Effects:** Evidence of decreased viral replication and reduced viral load with slowed progression of HIV and its sequelae.

Pharmacokinetics
Absorption: Well absorbed following oral administration.
Distribution: Unknown.
Metabolism and Excretion: Mostly metabolized by the uridine diphosphate glucuronosyltransferase (UGT) A1A enzyme system; 23% excreted in urine as parent drug and metabolite.
Half-life: 9 hr.

TIME/ACTION PROFILE (blood levels)

ROUTE	ONSET	PEAK	DURATION
PO	unknown	3 hr	12 hr

Contraindications/Precautions
Contraindicated in: OB: Lactation (breast feeding not recommended in HIV-infected patients).
Use Cautiously in: Geri: Choose dose carefully, considering concurrent disease states, drug therapy and age-related decrease in hepatic and renal function; Concurrent use of medications associated with rhabomyolysis/myopathy (may increase risk); **OB:** Use in pregnancy only if maternal benefit outweighs fetal risk; **Pedi:** Safe use in children <16 yr not established.

Adverse Reactions/Side Effects
CNS: headache, dizziness, fatigue, weakness. **CV:** myocardial infarction. **GI:** diarrhea, abdominal pain, gastritis, hepatitis, vomiting. **GU:** renal failure/impairment. **Hemat:** anemia, neutropenia. **Metab:** lipodystrophy. **Misc:** hypersensitivi-

ty reactions, immune reconstitution syndrome, fever.

Interactions
Drug-Drug: Concurrent use with **strong inducers of the UGT A1A enzyme system** including **rifampin** may ↓ blood levels and effectiveness. Concurrent use with **strong inhibitors of the UGT A1A enzyme system** may ↑ blood levels. ↑ risk of rhabomyolysis/myopathy **HMG-CoA reductase inhibitors**.

Route/Dosage
PO (Adults): 400 mg twice daily.

Availability
Tablets: 400 mg.

NURSING IMPLICATIONS

Assessment
- Assess patient for change in severity of HIV symptoms and for symptoms of opportunistic infections during therapy.
- *Lab Test Considerations:* Monitor viral load and CD4 counts regularly during therapy.
- May casue ↓ ANC, hemoglobin, and platelet counts.
- May cause ↑ serum glucose, AST, ALT, GGT, total bilirubin, alkaline phosphatase, pancreatic amylase, serum lipase, and creatinine kinase concentrations.

Potential Nursing Diagnoses
Risk for infection (Indications)
Noncompliance (Patient/Family Teaching)

Implementation
- **PO:** Must be administered without regard to meals.

Patient/Family Teaching
- Emphasize the importance of taking raltegravir as directed, at evenly spaced times throughout day. Do not take more than prescribed amount

and do not stop taking without consulting health care professional. If a dose is missed, take as soon as remembered unless almost time for next dose. Do not double doses. Advise patient to read Patient Information sheet before starting therapy and with each prescription renewal in chase changes have been made.

- Instruct patient that raltegravir should not be shared with others.
- Advise patient to avoid taking other Rx, OTC, or herbal products without consulting health care professional.
- Inform patient that raltegravir does not cure AIDS or prevent associated or opportunistic infections. Raltegravir does not reduce the risk of transmission of HIV to others through sexual contact or blood contamination. Caution patient to use a condom during sexual contact and to avoid sharing needles or donating blood to prevent spreading the AIDS virus to others. Advise patient that the long-term effects of raltegravir are unknown at this time.
- Advise patient to notify health care professional if they develop any unusual symptoms or if any known symptom persists or worsens.
- Advise patients to notify health care professional if pregnancy is planned or suspected. Breastfeeding should be avoided during therapy.
- Emphasize the importance of regular follow-up exams and blood counts to determine progress and monitor for side effects.

Evaluation/Desired Outcomes

- Delayed progression of AIDS and decreased opportunistic infections in patients with HIV.
- Decrease in viral load and improvement in CD4 cell counts.

rilonacept (ri-lon-a-sept)
Arcalyst
Classification
Thera: orphan drugs
Pharm: fusion proteins, interleukin antagonists

Pregnancy Category C

Indications

Treatment of Cryopyrin-Associated Periodic Syndromes (CAPS), including Familial Cold Autoinflammatory Syndrome (FCAS) and Muckle-Wells Syndrome (MWS).

Action

Modulates cryopyrin by blocking interleukin-1 beta (IL-1β) preventing its interaction with surface receptors. **Therapeutic Effects:** Decreased inflammatory manifestations of CAPS including fever, rash, arthralgia, myalgia, fatigue and conjunctivitis.

Pharmacokinetics

Absorption: Absorbed following subcutaneous administration.
Distribution: Unknown.
Metabolism and Excretion: Unknown.
Half-life: Unknown.

TIME/ACTION PROFILE (improvement in symptoms)

ROUTE	ONSET	PEAK	DURATION
Subcut	within several days	unknown	unknown

Contraindications/Precautions

Contraindicated in: Active or chronic infections; **OB:** May cause fetal harm.
Use Cautiously in: Patients at risk of infections; **Lactation:** Use cautiously; **Pedi:** Safety and effectiveness have not been established in children <12 yr.

Adverse Reactions/Side Effects

Resp: <u>upper respiratory tract infections</u>, cough. **Local:** <u>injection site reactions</u>. **Metab:** changes in lipid profile. **Neuro:** hypoesthesia. **Misc:** SERIOUS LIFE-THREATENING INFECTIONS, hypersensitivity reactions.

Interactions

Drug-Drug: May decrease the antibody response to and ↑ adverse reactions from **live vaccines**; vaccination should take place prior to initiation of treatment. Concurrent use with **TNF inhibitors** ↑ risk of serious infections and is not recommended. **Medications that are substrates of the CYP450 enzyme system**, especially those with narrow therapeutic indices such as **warfarin** should be monitored carefully as enzyme activity may increase (normalize) as a result of treatment.

Route/Dosage

Subcut: (Adults ≥ 18 yr): 320 mg initially, followed by 160 mg weekly.
Subcut: (Children and adolescents 12–17 yr): 4.4 mg/kg (not to exceed 320 mg) initially, followed by 2.2 mg/kg (not to exceed 160 mg) weekly.

Availability

Powder for subcutaneous administration (requires reconstitution): 220 mg/20 mL vial.

NURSING IMPLICATIONS

Assessment

- Assess for signs of infections. Discontinue therapy if serious infection occurs. Do not administer to patients with active or chronic infections.
- Assess for signs of hypersensitivity reactions; institute symptomatic therapy.
- *Lab Test Considerations:* Monitor lipid profiles every 2–3 months during therapy. May cause ↑ total cholesterol, HDL, LDL, and triglycerides. Consider lipid lowering therapies as needed.

Potential Nursing Diagnoses

Risk for infection (Adverse Reactions)

Implementation

- Administer all recommended adult and pediatric vaccinations, including pneumococcal vaccine and inactivated influenza vaccine, prior to starting rilonacept therapy.
- Administer first dose under supervision of health care professional.
- Loading dose in adults is given as two 2 mL injections on the same day in 2 different injection sites. In pediatric patients 1 or 2 injections may be used. Do not administer more than once weekly or more then 2 mL/injection site.
- Reconstitute with 2.3 mL of Sterile water for injection using a 27-gauge 1/2 inch needle for a concentration of 80 mg/mL. Discard needle and syringe after reconstitution. Shake vial for 1 min and allow to sit for 1 min. Solution is viscous, clear, colorless to pale yellow. Do not administer solutions that are discolored, contain particulate matter, or are passed the expiration date. Withdraw recommended dose up to 2 mL with new 27-gauge 1/2 inch needle. Vials are single use; discard unused solution. Rilonacept must be refrigerated and protected from light. Reconstituted solution is stable for 3 hrs at room temperature.
- **Subcut:** Inject subcut into abdomen (avoid area within 2 inches of navel), thigh or upper arm by pinching skin and injecting at a 90° (45° angle for small children or persons with little fat). May require 30 seconds to inject entire dose. Pull needle out of skin and hold gauze over

site for several seconds. Rotate sites and avoid sites that are bruised, red, tender or hard.

Patient/Family Teaching

- Instruct patient or family on correct technique for preparing and administering injection, and disposing of equipment. If a dose is missed, administer up to the day before next scheduled dose. Take next dose at regularly scheduled time. Advise patient to read *Patient Information* prior to starting therapy and with each Rx refill in case of new information.
- Advise patient to notify health care professional immediately if signs of infection (fever, cough, flu-like symptoms, open sores) occur during therapy.
- Instruct patient to notify health care professional or seek emergency care if signs of allergic reaction (rash, swollen face, difficulty breathing) occur.
- Advise patient that injection site reactions (erythema, swelling pruritus, bruising, inflammation, pain, edema, dermatitis, urticaria, vesicles, warmth, and hemorrhage) may occur; usually resolve in 1–2 days. Notify health care professional if reaction is persistent.
- Instruct patient to consult health care professional prior to taking other Rx, OTC, or herbal products.
- Advise female patients to notify health care professional if pregnancy is planned or suspected or if breastfeeding.

Evaluation/Desired Outcomes

- Decrease in symptoms (rash, joint pain, fever, tiredness), decrease in and normalization of serum Amyloid A (SAA) and C-Reactive Protein (CRP) levels.

romiplostim
(roe-mi-**ploss**-tim)
Nplate

Classification
Thera: Antithrombocytopenics
Pharm: thrombopoetin receptor agonists

Pregnancy Category C

Indications
Treatment of thrombocytopenia associated with chronic immune (idiopathic) thrombocytopenic purpura that has not responded to corticosteroids, immunoglobulins, or splenectomy where there is risk of bleeding.

Action
Acts as thrombopoetin (TPO) receptor agonist. **Therapeutic Effects:** Improved platelet count with decreased sequelae of thrombocytopenia (bleeding).

Pharmacokinetics
Absorption: Well absorbed following subcutaneous administration.
Distribution: Binds to specific cellular receptors.
Metabolism and Excretion: Unknown.
Half-life: 1–34 days.

TIME/ACTION PROFILE

ROUTE	ONSET	PEAK	DURATION
Subcut	unknown	1 wk	2 wk

Contraindications/Precautions
Contraindicated in: None noted;.
Use Cautiously in: Hepatic or renal impairment; **Geri:** Elderly patients may be more sensitive to effects, escalate dose cautiously, consider concurrent disease states, age-realtied decreases in organ function and drug therapy; **OB:** May cause fetal harm, enroll in

registry; avoid use during lactation; **Pedi:** Safe use in children <18 yr not established.

Adverse Reactions/Side Effects

CNS: dizziness, insomnia, headache. **GI:** abdominal pain, dyspepsia. **Hemat:** bone marrow fibrosis, thrombosis/thromboembolism (dose related). **MS:** extremity pain, myalgia, arthralgia, shoulder pain. **Neuro:** paresthesia.

Interactions

Drug-Drug: Drugs affecting platelet function should be avoided.

Route/Dosage

Subcut: (Adults): 1 mcg/kg weekly, increase by 1 mcg/kg weekly to achieve and maintain platelet count of $\geq 50 \times 10^9$/L up to 10 mcg/kg.

Availability

Single-use vial (requires reconstitution): 250 mcg, 500 mcg.

NURSING IMPLICATIONS

Assessment

- Assess for bruising and bleeding throughout therapy.
- *Lab Test Considerations:* Monitor CBC, including platelet counts and periperal blood smears, prior to, weekly until a stable platelet count ($\geq 50 \times 10^9$/L for 4 wks without dose adjustment) is achieved, and at least monthly thereafter. Do not administer if platelet count >400 $\times 10^9$/L. Continue monitoring for at least 2 wks following discontinuation. Discontinuation may result in worsened thrombocytopenia. Excessive doses may increase risk of thrombolic/thromboembolic complications.
- Monitor peripheral blood for signs of marrow fibrosis. Prior to initiation of therapy, establish baseline cellular morphologic abnormalities

and monitor monthly. If new or worsening abnormalities or cytopenia occur, discontinue romiplostim and consider bone marrow biopsy, including staining for fibrosis.
- If platelet counts decrease following initial response, assess for formation of neutralizing antibodies. May require submitting blood samples to Amgen (1-800-772-6436) for assay.

Potential Nursing Diagnoses

Risk for injury (Indications)

Implementation

- Romiplostim is available only through a restricted distribution program, the *Nplate NEXUS*. Only prescribers and patients registered with the program are able to prescribe, administer, and receive the product.
- Adjust dose based on platelet count. If platelet count is <50 $\times 10^9$/L, increase dose by 1 mcg/kg. If platelet count is >200 $\times 10^9$/L for 2 consecutive wks, reduce dose by 1 mcg/kg. If platelet count is >400 $\times 10^9$/L do not dose. Continue to assess platelet count weekly. After platelet count has fallen to <200 $\times 10^9$/L, resume romiplostim at a dose reduced by 1 mcg/kg.
- **Subcut:** Administer as a subcut injection once weekly. *Diluent:* Reconstitute 250 mcg vial with 0.72 mL and 500 mcg vial with 1.2 mL of preservative-free Sterile Water for Injection. *Concentration:* 500 mcg/mL. Gently swirl vial to reconstitute; do not shake. Dissolution usually takes less than 2 min. Injection volume may be very small; use syringe with graduations to 0.01 mL. Solution is clear and colorless; do not administer solutions that are discol-

ored or contain a precipitate. Protect solution from light. Reconstituted solution is stable at room temperature or if refrigerated for 24 hr. Discard unused portions of single-use vial. Do not administer more than one dose from each vial.

- Romiplostim may be used with other therapies such as corticosteroids, danazol, azathioprine, immunoglobulin IV, and anti-D immunoglobulin.

Patient/Family Teaching

- Explain *Nplate NEXUS* program to patient and assist with enrollment; risks associated with long-term administration are unknown. If a dose is missed, contact health care professional to arrange for next dose as soon as possible.
- Instruct patient to notify health care professional of any bruising or bleeding that occurs during therapy or of any side effects that are bothersome or do not go away.
- Advise patient to notify health care professional if pregnancy is planned or suspected. Inform pregnant patients of potential risks of therapy and encourage enrollment in pregnancy registry by calling 1-877-Nplate1. Romiplostim should not be used while breastfeeding.
- Advise patients to avoid situations or medications that may increase the risk of bleeding.
- Emphasize the importance or repeated lab tests.

Evaluation/Desired Outcomes

- Improved platelet count with decreased risk of bleeding. Discontinue if platelet count does not increase to a level sufficient to avoid clinically important bleeding after 4 wks at maximum weekly dose.

---

rufinamide (roo-fin-a-mide)
Banzol
Classification
Thera: anticonvulsants
Pharm: triazoles

Pregnancy Category C

Indications

Adjunctive treatment of seizures associated with Lennox-Gastaut syndrome in patients >4 yr.

Action

Although antiepileptic mechanism is unknown, rufinamide modulates the activity of sodium channels, prolonging the inactive state of the channel. **Therapeutic Effects:** Decreased incidence and severity of seizures associated with Lennox-Gastaut syndrome.

Pharmacokinetics

Absorption: 85% absorbed following oral administration; food enhances absorption.
Distribution: Evenly distributed between erythrocytes and plasma.
Metabolism and Excretion: Extensively metabolized; metabolites are primarily renaly excreted.
Half-life: 6–10 hr.

TIME/ACTION PROFILE

ROUTE	ONSET	PEAK	DURATION
PO	unknown	4–6 hr	12 hr

Contraindications/Precautions

Contraindicated in: Hypersensitivity; Familial Short QT syndrome; Severe hepatic impairment.
Use Cautiously in: History of suicidal thoughts or behavior; Mild to moderate hepatic impairment.

Adverse Reactions/Side Effects

CNS: dizziness, fatigue, headache, somnolence, ↑ suicidal thoughts/behavior.

EENT: diplopia. **CV:** QT prolongation. **GI:** <u>nausea</u>, changes in appetite. **GU:** urinary frequency. **Derm:** rash. **Hemat:** anemia. **Neuro:** ataxia, coordination abnormalities, gait disturbances. **Misc:** MULTI-ORGAN HYPERSENSITIVITY REACTIONS, hypersensitivity reactions (↑ children).

Interactions
Drug-Drug: Potent inducers of the CYP450 enzyme including **carbamazepine**, **phenytoin**, **primidone**, and **phenobarbital** ↑ clearance and may ↓ blood levels. **Valproate** ↓ clearance and may ↑ blood levels; valproate should be started at a low dose in patients stabilized on rufinamide. In patients stabilized on valproate, rufinamide should be started at a low dose. May ↓ blood levels and effectiveness of **hormonal contraceptives**. May ↑ blood levels of **phenytoin**.

Route/Dosage
PO (Adults): 400–800 mg/day in two divided doses, increase by 400–800 mg every 2 days until a maximum daily dose of 3200 mg/day (1600 mg twice daily) is reached.
PO (Children ≥ 4 yr): 10 mg/kg/day in two divided doses, increase by 10 mg/kg every 2 days until a maximum daily dose of 45 mg/kg/day or 3200 mg/day given in 2 divided doses, whichever is less, is reached.

Availability
Tablets: 200 mg.

NURSING IMPLICATIONS

Assessment
- Assess location, duration, and characteristics of seizure activity. Institute seizure precautions.
- Monitor closely for notable changes in behavior that could indicate the emergence or worsening of suicidal thoughts or behavior or depression.

- *Lab Test Considerations:* May cause leucopenia, anemia, neutropenia, and thrombocytopenia.

Potential Nursing Diagnoses
Risk for injury (Indications)

Implementation
- **PO:** Administer with food. Tablets can be cut in half for dosing flexibility. Tablets may be administered as whole or half tablets, or crushed.

Patient/Family Teaching
- Instruct patient to take rufinamide around the clock, as directed. Medication should be gradually discontinued over by 25% every 2 days to prevent seizures. Advise patient to read the *Medication Guide* before starting therapy and with each Rx refill.
- May cause drowsiness, dizziness, ataxia, and incoordination. Caution patient to avoid driving or other activities requiring alertness until response to medication is known. Tell patient not to resume driving until physician gives clearance based on control of seizure disorder.
- Inform patients and families of risk of suicidal thoughts and behavior and advise that behavioral changes, emergency or worsening signs and symptoms of depression, unusual changes in mood, or emergence of suicidal thoughts, behavior, or thoughts of self-harm should be reported to health care professional immediately.
- Instruct patient to notify health care professional if signs of multiorgan hypersensitivity reactions (fever, rash, fatigue, jaundice, dark urine) occur.
- Advise patient to consult health care professional before taking other Rx, OTC, or herbal preparations and to avoid taking alcohol or other CNS

depressants concurrently with rufinamide.

- Advise female patients to notify health care professional if pregnancy is planned or suspected or if breastfeeding. Use of rufinamide decreases effectiveness of oral contraceptives. Advise patient to use a non-hormonal method of contraception during therapy.

Evaluation/Desired Outcomes
- Decreased frequency and intensity of seizure activity.

---

sapropterin (sa-**prop**-te-rin)
Kuvan
Classification
Thera: antihyperphenylalaninemics
Pharm: synthetic BH4

Pregnancy Category C

Indications
To reduce phenylalanine (Phe) levels in patients with hyperphenylalaninemia (HPA) caused by tetrahydrobiopterin-(BH4−) responsive phenylketonuria (PKU); used with a Phe-restricted diet.

Action
Acts as a synthetic form of the cofactor (BH4) for the enzyme phenylalanine hydoxylase (PAH). PAH converts phenylalanine to tyrosine. In PKU patients, activity of PAH is deficient. BH4 helps to activate PAH and thus reduce Phe levels. **Therapeutic Effects:** Preservation of brain function by lowering Phe levels.

Pharmacokinetics
Absorption: Well absorbed following oral administration; food increases absorption.
Distribution: Unknown.
Metabolism and Excretion: Unknown.

Half-life: 6.7 hr.

TIME/ACTION PROFILE (effect on Phe levels)

ROUTE	ONSET	PEAK	DURATION
PO	within 24 hr	up to one mo	unknown

Contraindications/Precautions
Contraindicated in: Lactation: Should not be used if breast feeding.
Use Cautiously in: Hepatic or renal impairment; Concurrent use of levodopa; **OB:** Use during pregnancy only if clearly needed; **Pedi:** Safety and effectiveness in children <4 yr not established.

Adverse Reactions/Side Effects
CNS: headache. **EENT:** pharyngolaryngeal pain. **GI:** abdominal pain, diarrhea, nausea, vomiting. **Hemat:** neutropenia.

Interactions
Drug-Drug: Concurrent use of **medications known to inhibit folate metabolism** including **methotrexate** can ↓ BH4 levels; use cautiously. Concurrent use of **medications known to affect nitric oxide-mediated vasorelaxation** including **sildenafil**, **vardenafil**, or **tadalafil** could ↑ risk of hypotension. Concurrent use of **levodopa** may ↑ risk of seizures, over-stimulation and irritatibility; use cautiously.

Route/Dosage
PO (Adults): 10 mg/kg once daily, titrated on the basis of Phe levels (range 5–20mg/kg/day).

Availability
Tablets: 100 mg.

NURSING IMPLICATIONS
Assessment
- Assess diet prior to and during therapy. Provide nutritional counseling. All patients with PKU should main-

---

tain a Phe-restricted diet. During dose titration, dietary Phe intake must remain stable to determine effectiveness of sapropterin.

- Monitor for signs of allergic reaction (rash).
- ***Lab Test Considerations:*** Monitor blood Phe levels after 1 wk of treatment and periodically for up to 1 month. If blood Phe does not decrease from baseline at 10 mg/kg/day dose after 1 wk, may increase to 20 mg/kg/day. Patients whose blood Phe does not decrease within 1 month of treatment with 20 mg/kg/day dose are considered non-responders and therapy should be discontinued. Prolonged elevations of Phe in patients with PKU can result in neurologic damage including mental retardation, microcephaly, delayed speech, seizures, and behavioral abnormalities. Prolonged levels that are too low can cause catabolism and protein breakdown.

Potential Nursing Diagnoses
Imbalanced nutrition: more than body requirements (Indications)
Deficient knowledge, related to diet and medication regimen (Patient/Family Teaching)

Implementation
- **PO:** Administer with food to increase absorption. Dissolve tablets in 4–8 oz of water or apple juice and administer within 15 min of dissolution. Tablets may take several minutes to dissolve; stirring or crushing tablets may make dissolution faster. Small pieces floating on top of water or apple juice are normal and safe for patients to swallow. If small pieces remain in glass after drinking medicine, add more water or apple juice to make sure complete dose is administered. Protect tablets from moisture, do not remove dessicant

packet. Color of tablets may change over time to light yellow; this is normal and tablets are safe. Do not use tablets that have expired.

Patient/Family Teaching
- Instruct patient to take saropterin as directed at the same time each day. Take missed doses as soon as remembered that day; do not take 2 doses in the same day, omit dose if remembered next day. Instruct patient to read the *Patient Information* guide prior to taking sapropterin and with each Rx refill, in case of new information.
- Advise patient to avoid making changes to dietary PhE without consulting health care professional; any dietary changes may affect Phe level.
- Instruct patient to notify health care professional if fever or illness occurs; dose may need to be adjusted.
- Advise patient to consult health care professional prior to taking other Rx, OTC, or herbal products.
- Advise female patients to notify health care professional if pregnancy is planned or suspected or if breastfeeding.

Evaluation/Desired Outcomes
- Reduction of Phe levels.

---

silodosin (si-lo-do-sin)
Rapaflo
Classification
Thera: benign prostatic hyperplasia (BPH) agents
Pharm: alpha-adrenergic blockers

Pregnancy Category B

Indications
Treatment of the signs/symptoms or Benign Prostatic Hyperplasia (BPH).

Action
Blocks post synaptic alpha₁ -adrenergic receptors. Decreases contractions in the smooth muscle of the prostatic capsule. **Therapeutic Effects:** Decreased signs and symptoms of BPH (urinary urgency, hesitancy, nocturia).

Pharmacokinetics
Absorption: 32% absorbed following oral administration.
Distribution: Unknown.
Protein Binding: 97%.
Metabolism and Excretion: Extensively metabolized (CYP3A4, UGT2B7 and other metabolic pathways involved); 33.5% excreted in urine and 54.9% in feces.
Half-life: 13.3 hr.

TIME/ACTION PROFILE (effect on symptoms of BPH)

ROUTE	ONSET	PEAK	DURATION
PO	rapid	24 hr	24 hr*

*Following discontinuation.

Contraindications/Precautions
Contraindicated in: Not indicated for use in women or children; Severe renal impairment (CrCl less than 30 mL/min); Severe hepatic impairment (Child-Pugh score of 10 or greater); Concurrent use of strong CYP3A4 inhibitors or P-gp inhibitors.
Use Cautiously in: Moderate inhibitors of the CYP3A4 enzyme system; Cataract surgery (may cause Intraoperative Floppy Iris Syndrome); Moderate renal impairment (lower dose recommended); **Geri:** Increased risk of orthostatic hypotention; **Pedi:** Safety and effectiveness have not been established.

Adverse Reactions/Side Effects
CNS: dizziness, headache. **CV:** orthostatic hypotension. **GI:** diarrhea. **GU:** <u>retrograde ejaculation</u>.

Interactions
Drug-Drug: Strong inhibitors of CYP3A4 (including **ketoconazole, clarithromycin, itraconazole,** and **ritonavir**) ↓ metabolism, ↑ blood levels and risk of toxicity; concurrent use is contraindicated. Concurrent use with **moderate CYP3A4 inhibitors** (including **diltiazem, erythromycin,** and **verapamil**) may ↑ silodosin levels; use cautiously. Concurrent use with **antihypertensives** (including **calcium channel blockers** and **thiazides**), other **alpha blockers** and **phosphodiesterase type 5 inhibitors** (including **sildenafil** and **tadalafil**) ↑ the risk of dizziness and orthostatic hypotension. **P-glycoprotein (P-gp) inhibitors** including **cyclosporine**) may ↑ levels; concurrent use not recommended.

Route/Dosage
PO (Adults): 8 mg once daily **Renal Impairment**
PO (Adults CCr 30–50 mL/min): 4 mg once daily.

Availability
Capsules: 4 mg, 8 mg.

NURSING IMPLICATIONS

Assessment
- Assess patient for symptoms of benign prostatic hyperplasia (urinary hesitancy, feeling of incomplete bladder emptying, interruption of urinary stream, impairment of size and force of urinary stream, terminal urinary dribbling, straining to start flow, frequency, dysuria, nocturia, urgency) before and periodically during therapy.
- Assess patient for orthostatic reaction and syncope. Monitor BP (lying and standing) and during initial therapy and periodically thereafter.
- Rule out prostatic carcinoma before therapy; symptoms are similar.

Potential Nursing Diagnoses
Risk for injury (Side Effects)
Noncompliance (Patient/Family
Teaching)

Implementation
- **PO:** Administer with food at the
same meal each day.

Patient/Family Teaching
- Instruct patient to take medication
with the same meal each day.
- May cause dizziness. Caution patient
to avoid driving or other activities requiring alertness until response to
the medication is known.
- Caution patient to avoid sudden
changes in position to decrease orthostatic hypotension, especially patients with low blood pressure or
concurrently taking
antihypertensives.
- Advise patient to consult health care
professional before taking any other
Rx, OTC, or herbal products, especially cough, cold, or allergy
remedies.
- Instruct patient to notify health care
professional of medication regimen
before any surgery. Patients plan-
ning cataract surgery should notify
opthalmologist of silodosin therapy
prior to surgery.
- Inform patient that silodosin may
cause retrograde ejaculation (or-
gasm with reduced or no semen).
This does not pose a safety concern
and is reversible with
discontinuation.
- Emphasize the importance of follow-
up exams to evaluate effectiveness of
medication.
- **Geri:** Assess risk for falls; imple-
ment fall prevention program and
instruct patient and family in preventing falls at home.

Evaluation/Desired Outcomes
- Decreased symptoms of benign
prostatic hyperplasia.

---

tapentadol (ta-pen-ta-dol)
Nucynta
Classification
Thera: analgesics (centrally
acting), opioid analgesics
Pharm: opioid agonists

Schedule II

Pregnancy Category C

Indications
Management of moderate to severe
acute pain in patients ≥18 yr.

Action
Acts as μ-opioid receptor agonist. Also
inhibits the reuptake of norepinephrine. **Therapeutic Effects:** Decrease
in pain severity.

Pharmacokinetics
Absorption: 32% absorbed following
oral administration.
Distribution: Widely distributed.
Metabolism and Excretion: Under-
goes extensive first-pass hepatic metabolism (97%); metabolites have no analgesic activity; metabolized drug is
99% renally excreted.
Half-life: 4 hr.

TIME/ACTION PROFILE (analgesic
effect)

ROUTE	ONSET	PEAK	DURATION
PO	unknown	1 hr	4–6 hr

Contraindications/Precautions
Contraindicated in: Significant respiratory depression in unmonitored settings or where resuscitative equipment
is not readily available; Paralytic ileus;
Severe hepatic impairment; Concurrent

MAO inhibitors or use of MAO inhibitors in the preceding 2 wk; **Lactation:** Lactation; **Pedi:** Safe use in children <18 yr not established; not recommended.

Use Cautiously in: Conditions associated with hypoxia, hypercapnea, or decreased respiratory reserve including asthma, chronic obstructive pulmonary disease, cor pulmonale, extreme obesity, sleep apnea syndrome, myxedema, kyphoscoliosis, CNS depression, use of other CNS depressants or coma (↑ risk of further respiratory depression); use smallest effective dose; **Geri:** Elderly or debilitated patients (↑ risk of respiratory depression); consider age-related decrease in hepatic, renal and cardiovascular function, concurrent disease states and drug therapy (initial dose should be lower); History of substance abuse or addiction disorder; History or ↑ risk of seizures; **OB:** Use in pregnancy only if potential benefit justifies potential risk to the fetus.

Adverse Reactions/Side Effects

CNS: SEIZURES, dizziness, headache, somnolence. **Resp:** RESPIRATORY DEPRESSION. **GI:** nausea, vomiting.

Interactions

Drug-Drug: Concurrent **MAO inhibitors** or use of MAO inhibitors in the preceding 2 wk can result in potentially life-threatening adverse cardiovascular reactions due to additive effects on norepinephrine levels. Concurrent use of other **CNS depressants** including **sedative/hypnotics**, **alcohol**, **antihistamines**, **antidepressants**, **phenothiazines**, and other **opioids** ↑ risk of further CNS depression; consider dose ↓ of one or both agents. ↑ risk of serotonin syndrome with **SNRIs**, **SSRIs**, **triptans**, **tricyclic antidepressants**, and **MAO inihibitors**.

Route/Dosage

PO (Adults): 50, 75, or 100 mg initially, then every 4–6 hr as needed and tolerated. If pain control is not achieved within first hour of first dose, additional dose may be given. Doses should not exceed 700 mg on the first day or 600 mg/day thereafter

Hepatic Impairment

PO (Adults): *Moderate hepatic impaitment*—50 mg every 8 hr initially, then titrate to maintain analgesia without intolerable side effects.

Availability

Immediate-release tablets: 50 mg, 75mg, 100 mg.

NURSING IMPLICATIONS

Assessment

- Assess type, location, and intensity of pain before and 1 hr (peak) after administration.
- Assess blood pressure and respiratory rate before and periodically during administration. Monitor for respiratory depression especially during initial dosing and with patients at increased risk.
- Assess bowel function routinely. Prevention of constipation should be instituted with increased intake of fluids and bulk and with laxatives to minimize constipating effects. Administer stimulant laxatives routinely if opioid use exceeds 2–3 days, unless contraindicated.
- Prolonged use may lead to physical and psychological dependence and tolerance, although these may be milder than with opioids. This should not prevent patient from receiving adequate analgesia. Most patients who receive tapentadol for pain do not develop psychological dependence.
- Monitor patient for seizures. May occur within recommended dose

range. Risk is increased in patients with a history of seizures and in patients taking antidepressants (SSRIs, SNRIs, tricyclics) or other drugs that decrease the seizure threshold.

- Monitor for serotonin syndrome (mental-status changes [agitation, hallucinations, coma], autonomic instability [tachycardia, labile blood pressure, hyperthermia], neuromuscular aberrations [hyperreflexia, incoordination] and/or gastrointestinal symptoms [nausea, vomiting, diarrhea] in patients taking these drugs concurrently.
- *Toxicity and Overdose:* Overdose may cause respiratory depression. Naloxone (Narcan) may reverse some, but not all, of the symptoms of overdose. Treatment should be symptomatic and supportive. Maintain adequate respiratory exchange.

Potential Nursing Diagnoses
Acute pain (Indications)

Implementation
- Initial dose of 50 mg, 75 mg, or 100 mg is individualized based on pain severity, previous experience with similar drugs, and ability to monitor patient. Second dose may be administered as soon as 1 hr after first dose if adequate pain relief is not obtained with first dose.
- **PO:** Tapentadol may be administered without regard to meals.

Patient/Family Teaching
- Instruct patient on how and when to ask for pain medication and to take tapentadol as directed; do not adjust dose without consulting health care professional. Report breakthrough pain and adverse reactions to health care professional. Do not take tapentadol if pain is mild or can be controlled with other pain medications such as NSAIDs or acetaminophen. Do not stop abruptly; may cause withdrawal symptoms (anxiety, sweating, insomina, rigors, pain, nausea, tremors, diarrhea, upper respiratory symptoms, hallucinations). Decrease dose gradually. Advise patient to read the *Medication Guide* prior to taking tapentadol and with each Rx refill, in case of new information.
- Do not share tapentadol with others, even it they have the same symptoms; may be dangerous.
- May cause dizziness and drowsiness. Caution patient to avoid driving or other activities requiring alertness until response to medication is known.
- Inform patient that tapentadol may cause seizures. Stop taking tapentadol and notify health care professional immediately if seizures occur.
- Advise patient to change positions slowly to minimize orthostatic hypotension.
- Caution patient to avoid concurrent use of alcohol or other CNS depressants with this medication.
- Advise patient to consult health care professional before taking other RX, OTC, or herbal products concurrently.
- Advise patient to notify health care professional if signs or serotonin syndrome occur.
- **OB:** Advise female patients to notify health care professional if pregnancy is planned or suspected, or if breastfeeding.
- Encourage patient to turn, cough, and breathe deeply every 2 hr to prevent atelectasis.

Evaluation/Desired Outcomes
- Decrease in severity of pain without a significant alteration in level of consciousness or respiratory status.

temsirolimus
(tem-si-**ro**-li-mus)
Torisel
Classification
Thera: antineoplastics
Pharm: enzyme inhibitors, kinase inhibitors

Pregnancy Category D

Indications
Advanced renal cell carcinoma.

Action
Binds to an intracellular protein. The resultant complex inhibits an enzyme, mTOR (mammalian target of rapamycin). Inhibition of this enzyme arrests cell growth in the G1 phase. **Therapeutic Effects:** Decreased spread of renal cell carcinoma.

Pharmacokinetics
Absorption: IV administration results in complete bioavailability.
Distribution: Temsirolimus and sirolimus partition extensively in formed blood elements.
Metabolism and Excretion: Mostly metabolized by the liver to sirolimus, an active metabolite Primarily eliminated in feces.
Half-life: *Temsirolimus*—17.3 hr; *sirolimus*—54.6 hr.

TIME/ACTION PROFILE

ROUTE	ONSET	PEAK	DURATION
IV	unknown	end of infusion	1 wk

Contraindications/Precautions
Contraindicated in: OB: Pregnancy and lactation.
Use Cautiously in: Hypersensitivity to temsirolimus, sirolimus or polysorbate 80; Perioperative patients (may impair wound healing); **OB:** Patients which

child-bearing potential; **Pedi:** Safe use in children not established.

Adverse Reactions/Side Effects
CNS: weakness. **EENT:** conjunctivitis. **CV:** hypertension, venous thromboembolism. **Resp:** INTERSTITIAL LUNG DISEASE. **GI:** BOWEL PERFORATION, anorexia, ↑ liver enzymes, mucositis, nausea. **GU:** RENAL FAILURE. **Derm:** rash, abnormal wound healing. **Endo:** hyperglycemia. **F and E:** edema, hypophosphatemia. **Hemat:** anemia, leukopenia, lymphopenia, thrombocytopenia. **Metab:** hyperlipidemia, hypertriglyceridemia. **Misc:** hypersensitivity reactions including ANAPHYLAXIS, ↑ risk of infections.

Interactions
Drug-Drug: Concurrent use of strong **CYP3A4 enzyme inhibitors** including **ketoconazole, itraconozole, voriconazole, clarithromycin, telithromycin, atazanavir, indinavir, nelfinavir, ritonavir, saquinavir** ↑ blood levels and ↑ risk of toxicity; consider ↓ dose to 12.5 mg weekly. Concurrent use of strong **inducers of the CYP 3A4 enzyme system** including **dexamethasone, phenytoin, phenobarbital, carbamazepine, rifampin, rifabutin** or **rifampacin** may ↓ blood levels and ↓ efficacy; consider ↑ dose to 50 mg weekly. Concurrent use with **sunitinib** ↑ risk of toxicity (rash, gout, cellulitis). May ↓ antibody response to and ↑ risk of adverse reactions from **live virus vaccines**; avoid current use.
Drug-Natural Products: *St. John's wort* may ↓ blood levels; avoid concurrent use.
Drug-Food: **Grapefruit juice** may ↑ blood levels and ↑ risk of toxicity.

Route/Dosage
IV (Adults): 25 mg once weekly; dose modification is required for bone marrow toxicity or concurrent use of

agents affecting the CYP 3A4 enzyme system (pre-treatment with antihistamine is recommended).

Availability

Concentrated solution for IV infusion (must be diluted): 25 mg/1 ml in 1 ml vial (comes with a diluent containing polysorbate 80, polyethylene glycol 400 and dehydrated alcohol).

NURSING IMPLICATIONS

Assessment

- Assess for signs of hypersensitivity reactions (anaphylaxis, dyspnea, flushing, chest pain) during administration. If reaction occurs, stop infusion and observe patient for at least 30–60 min. May resume treatment with administration of an antihistamine (if not previously administered) and/or an H2 antagonist (such as IV famotidine 20 mg or IV ranitidine 50 mg) 30 min before restarting temsirolimus. Infuse at a slower rate over 60 min.
- Monitor for signs of infection, including opportunistic infection (sore throat; appearance of sputum, urine, stool; vital signs) during therapy.
- Monitor for signs of interstitial lung disease (dyspnea, cough, hypoxia, fever). May require discontinuation of therapy and/or treatment with corticosteroids and/or antibiotics.
- **Lab Test Considerations:** Monitor CBC and platelet count prior to and during therapy. May cause ↓ ANC and platelets. Hold dose if ANC <1000/mm³, platelet count <75,000/mm³, or adverse reactions grade 3 or greater. Once toxicities have resolved to grade 2 or less, may restart temsirolimus at a dose decreased by 5 mg/wk to a dose no lower than 15 mg/wk. May cause

↓ hemoglobin, lymphocytes, and leukocytes.
- Monitor serum glucose prior to and periodically during therapy. May cause ↓ serum glucose requiring increase in dose of or initiation of insulin or oral hypoglycemia agent therapy.
- Monitor serum cholesterol and triglycerides prior to and during therapy. May cause increase requiring initiation or increase in dose of lipid lowering agents.
- Monitor liver enzymes prior to and during therapy. May cause ↑ AST, alkaline phosphatase, serum creatine, and total bilirubin. May cause ↓ serum phosphorous and potassium.

Potential Nursing Diagnoses

Risk for infection (Adverse Reactions)

Implementation

- Premedicate with IV diphenhydramine 25–50 mg (or similar antihistamine) 30 min before start of each dose of temsirolimus.

IV Administration

- **Diluent:** Inject 1.8 mL of *diluent for Torisel* into temsirolimus vial for a concentration of 10 mg/mL. **Concentration:** Vial contains an overfill and total volume will be 3 mL of 10 mg/mL solution. Mix well by inversion of vial. Allow sufficient time for air bubbles to subside. Solution should be clear to slightly turbid, colorless to yellow, and free from visual particles.Store undiluted solution in refrigerator and protect from light during storage and preparation. Diluted solution is stable for 24 hr at room temperature. Withdraw required amount of temsirolimus 10 mg/mL solution and inject rapidly into 250 mL container (glass, polyolefin, or polyethylene) of 0.9% NaCl.

Mix by inversion; avoid excessive shaking to prevent foaming. Administer with non-DEHP (di-(2–ethylhexyl) phthalate tubing and an in-line filter with pore size of not >5 microns. *Rate:* Administer over 30–60 min using an infusion pump to ensure accurate delivery. Complete infusion within 6 hrs of mixture with 0.9% NaCl.

- **Y-Site Incompatibility:** Do not mix in solution or administer via Y-site with other solutions or medications.

Patient/Family Teaching

- Advise patient to notify health care professional immediately if any new or worsening abdominal pain or blood in stools occur or if signs of bowel perforation (fever, abdominal pain, metabolic acidosis, bloody stools, diarrhea) occur.
- Advise patient to avoid drinking grapefruit juice while taking temsirolimus.
- Advise patients to notify health care professional if excessive thirst or volume or frequency of urination and diabetic patients to closely monitor glucose.
- Inform patient of the increased risk for intracerebral bleeding with temsirolimus.
- Advise patient to consult health care professional prior to taking any Rx, OTC, or herbal products, especially St. John's Wort.
- Instruct patient not to receive any vaccinations without advice of health care professional and to avoid contact with persons who have received live vaccines during therapy.
- Advise female patients to avoid becoming pregnant during and for 3 mo after therapy. Men with partners of child-bearing potential should use reliable contraception throughout

therapy and for 3 mo after last dose of temsirolimus.

Evaluation/Desired Outcomes

- Decreased spread of renal cell carcinoma.

---

tetrabenazine
(te-tra-**ben**-a-zeen)
Xenazine

Classification
Thera: antichoreas
Pharm: reversible monoamine depleters

Pregnancy Category C

Indications

Treatment of chorea due to Huntington's Disease.

Action

Acts as a reversible inhibitor of the vesicle monoamine transporter type 2 (VMAT-2) which inhibits the reuptake of serotonin, norepinephrine and dopamine into vesicles in presynaptic neurons. **Therapeutic Effects:** Decreased chorea due to Huntington's Disease.

Pharmacokinetics

Absorption: At least 75% absorbed following oral administration.
Distribution: Crosses the blood-brain barrier.
Metabolism and Excretion: Rapidly and extensively metabolized by the liver; CYP2D6 plays a large role in the metabolic process. Metabolites are renally excreted. Two metabolites α-dihydrotetrabenazine (α- HTBZ) and β-HTBZ bind to VMAT-2 and are pharmacologically active.
Half-life: α-HTBZ- 4-8 hrs; β-HTBZ - 2-4 hr.

TIME/ACTION PROFILE (blood levels)

ROUTE	ONSET	PEAK	DURATION
PO	unknown	1.0–1.5 hr	12–18 hr*

*Return of symptoms following discontinuation.

Contraindications/Precautions

Contraindicated in: Hepatic impairment; Concurrent use of reserpine or MAO inhibitors; Patients who are actively suicidal or have untreated depression; **Lactation:** Breast feeding.
Use Cautiously in: History of/propensity for depression or history of psychiatric illness; history of suicidality; Poor CYP2D6 metabolizers; initial dose reduction required; Concurrent use of CYP2D6 inhibitors; dose modification required; Recent history of myocardial infarction or unstable heart disease; **OB:** Use during pregnancy only when potential benefit justifies potential risk to the fetus; **Pedi:** Safe and effective use in children has not been established.

Adverse Reactions/Side Effects

CNS: <u>anxiety</u>, <u>fatigue</u>, <u>insomnia</u>, <u>depression</u>, <u>sedation/somnolence</u>, cognitive defects, dizziness, headache. **Resp:** shortness of breath. **CV:** hypotension, QTc prolongation. **GI:** <u>nausea</u>, dysphagia. **Neuro:** <u>akathisia</u>, balance difficulty, dysarthria, parkinsonism, unsteady gait. **Misc:** NEUROLEPTIC MALIGNANT SYNDROME.

Interactions

Drug-Drug: Blood levels are ↑ by drugs that inhibit the CYP2D6 enzyme system including **fluoxetine**, **paroxetine**, and **quinidine**; initial dose reduction of tetrabenazine recommended. **Reserpine** binds to VMAT-2 and depletes monoamines in the CNS; avoid concurrent use; wait 3 wk after discontinuing to initiate tetrabenazine. Concurrent use of **MAO inhibitors** ↑ risk of serious adverse reactions and is contraindicated. Concurrent use with **neurolpetic drugs** or **dopamine antagonists** including **haloperidol**, **chlorpromazine**, **risperidone**, and **olanzapine** may ↑ risk of QTc prolongation, neuroleptic malignant syndrome and extrapyramidal disorders. Concurrent use of **alcohol** or other **CNS depressants** may ↑ risk of CNS depression.

Route/Dosage

PO (Adults): 12.5 mg/day for one wk initially, increased by 12.5 weekly up to 37.5–50 mg/day in three divided doses; *concurrent use of strong inhibitors or CYP2D6 or poor CYP2D6 metabolizers*—start with initial dose of 6.25 mg, titrate carefully.

Availability

Tablets: 12.5 mg, 25 mg.

NURSING IMPLICATIONS

Assessment

- Assess signs of Huntington's disease (changes in mood, cognition, chorea, rigidity, and functional capacity) periodically during therapy. Reevaluate need for tetrabenazine periodically by assessing beneficial effect and side effects; determination may require dose reduction or discontinuation. Underlying chorea may improve over time, decreasing need for tetrabenazine.
- Monitor closely for new or worsening depression or suicidality. If depression or suicidality occurs decrease dose and may initiate or increase dose of antidepressants.
- Monitor for signs of neuroleptic malignant syndrome (hyperpyrexia, muscle rigidity, altered mental status, irregular pulse or blood pressure, tachycardia, diaphoresis, cardiac dysrhythmia) periodically during therapy. If symptoms occur dis-

continue tetrabenazine and manage symptomatically. If re-introduction of tetrabenazine is considered monitor carefully; recurrences of neuroleptic malignant syndrome have occurred.

- Monitor patient for onset of akathisia (restlessness or desire to keep moving) and parkinsonian (difficulty speaking or swallowing, loss of balance control, pill rolling of hands, mask-like face, shuffling gait, rigidity, tremors). Notify health care professional if these symptoms occur; reduction in dose or discontinuation may be necessary.

- Monitor for tardive dyskinesia (uncontrolled rhythmic movement of mouth, face, and extremities; lip smacking or puckering; puffing of cheeks; uncontrolled chewing; rapid or worm-like movements of tongue, excessive eye blinking). Report these symptoms immediately; may be irreversible and reqquire discontinuation of therapy.

- Assess blood pressure sitting and standing. May cause orthostatic hypotension.

- ***Lab Test Considerations:*** Test for the CYP2D6 gene in patients requiring doses of >50 mg/day to determine if they are poor, intermediate, or extensive metabolizers. Limit dose to 50 mg in patients who are poor metabolizers.

Potential Nursing Diagnoses

Risk for suicide (Adverse Reactions)

Implementation

- Dose should be titrated slowly and individualized.

- **PO:** May be administered without regard to food.

Patient/Family Teaching

- Instruct patient to take tetrabenazine as directed. Do not take more or stop taking tetrabenazine without consulting health care professional. Dose adjustment may take several wk. Discuss procedure for missed doses with health care professional before beginning therapy; do not double doses. If a dose is missed or medication discontinued, involuntary movements will return or worsen in 12–18 hrs. If tetrabenazine is stopped for more than 5 days, consult health care professional before taking another dose; lower dose may be required.

- Advise patient and family to monitor for changes, especially sudden changes, in mood, behaviors, thoughts or feelings. If new or worse feelings of sadness or crying spells, lack of interest in friends or activities, sleeping a lot more or less, feelings of unimportance, guilt, hopelessness or helplessness, irritability or aggression, more or less hungry, difficulty paying attention, or thoughts of hurting self or ending life occur, notify health care professional promptly.

- Causes sedation. Caution patient to avoid driving and other activities requiring alertness until response to medication is known.

- Advise patient to avoid alcohol and other CNS depressants during therapy; increases sedation.

- Inform patient of potential side effects and instruct to notify health care professional if side effects occur.

- Advise patient to consult health care professional before taking other Rx, OTC, or herbal products.

- Advise female patients to notify health care professional if pregnancy is planned or suspected or if breastfeeding.

Evaluation/Desired Outcomes

- Decrease in chorea due to Huntington's disease.

---

trimipramine
(trye-**mip**-ra-meen)
Surmontil

Classification
Thera: antidepressants
Pharm: tricyclic antidepressants

Pregnancy Category C

Indications

Treatment of depression, often in conjunction with psychotherapy.

Action

Potentiates the effect of serotinin and norepinephrine in the CNS. Has significant anticholinergic properties, including sedation. **Therapeutic Effects:** Antidepressant action.

Pharmacokinetics

Absorption: Well absorbed following oral administration.
Distribution: Unknown.
Metabolism and Excretion: Mostly metabolized by the liver.
Half-life: 7–30 hr.

TIME/ACTION PROFILE

ROUTE	ONSET	PEAK	DURATION
PO	2–3 wk (up to 30 days)	2–6 wk	days–wks

Contraindications/Precautions

Contraindicated in: Hypersensitivity; cross-sensitivity may occur with other tricyclic antidepressants; Recovery phase following MI; Concurrent MAO inhibitor therapy; wait 2 wk following cessation to initiate trimipramine in lower doses initially; Angle-closure glaucoma.
Use Cautiously in: History or symptoms compatible with bipolar disease (may precipitate mixed/manic episodes; May ↑ risk of suicide attempt/ ideation especially during early treatment or dose adjustment; **Pedi:** risk may be greater in children and adolescents; Prostatic hyperplasia (↑ risk of urinary retention); History of seizures (may ↓ threshold); Hepatic impairment; Electroshock therapy (may ↑ risk of adverse reactions); Increased intraocular pressure; Hyperthyroidism (↑ risk of cardiovascular toxicity); **OB:** Use only if clearly needed and maternal benefits outweigh risks to fetus; **Lactation:** May cause sedation in infant; **Pedi:** Safety not established; **Geri:** ↑ risk of adverse reactions, including falls secondary to sedative and anticholinergic affects.
Exercise Extreme Caution in: Preexisting cardiovascular disease.

Adverse Reactions/Side Effects

CNS: lethargy,, sedation.. **EENT:** blurred vision, dry eyes, dry mouth. **CV:** ARRHYTHMIAS,, hypotension, ECG changes. **GI:** constipation, hepatitis, paralytic ileus, increased appetite, weight gain.. **GU:** urinary retention,, ↓ libido.. **Derm:** photosensitivity. **Endo:** changes in blood glucose, gynecomastia. **Hemat:** blood dyscrasias.

Interactions

Drug-Drug: Concurrent **MAO inhibitors** may result in hyperpyretic reactions, convulsive crises, and death. **Guanethidine or similar agents** (ef-

fects may be negated by trimipramine). Trimipramine is metabolized in the liver by the cytochrome P450 2D6 enzyme, and its action may be affected by drugs that compete for metabolism by this enzyme, including **other antidepressants**, **phenothiazines**, **carbamazepine**, **class 1C antiarrhythmics** including **propafenone**, and **flecainide**; when used concurrently dose of one or the other or both may be necessary. Concurrent use of other drugs that inhibit the activity of the enzyme, including **cimetidine**, **quinidine**, **amiodarone**, and **ritonavir**, may result in ↑ effects of trimipramine. Concurrent use with **SSRI antidepressants** may result in toxicity and should be avoided (fluoxetine should be stopped 5 wk before starting trimipramine). Concurrent use with **clonidine** may result in hypertensive crisis and should be avoided. Concurrent use with **levodopa** may result in delayed or absorption of levodopa or hypertension. Blood levels and effects may be ↓ by **rifamycins** (**rifampin**, **rifapentine**, and **rifabutin**). Concurrent use with **moxifloxacin** ↑ risk of adverse cardiovascular reactions. ↑ CNS depression with other **CNS depressants** including **alcohol**, **antihistamines**, **clonidine**, **opioids**, and **sedative/hypnotics**. **Barbiturates** may alter blood levels and effects. ↑ Adrenergic and anticholinergic side effects with other **agents having adrenergic or anticholinergic properties**. Levels and risk of toxicity may be ↑ by **phenothiazines** or **oral contraceptives**. Nicotine may ↑ metabolism and alter effects.
Drug-Natural Products: *St. John's wort* may ↓ serum concentrations and efficacy. Concomitant use of *kava*, *valerian*, or *chamomile* can ↑ CNS depression. ↑ anticholinergic effects with *jimson weed* and *scopolia*.

Route/Dosage
PO (Adults): 75 mg/day in divided doses or as a single daily dose at bedtime; may be increased up to 150 mg/day; not to exceed 200 mg/day (300 mg/day in hospitalized patients). *Adolescent and elderly patients*—50 mg/day, may gradually increase up to 100 mg/day.

Availability
capsules: 25 mg, 50 mg, 100 mg.

NURSING IMPLICATIONS
Assessment
- Monitor blood pressure and pulse before and during initial therapy. Notify health care professional of decreases in blood pressure (10–20 mmHg) or sudden increase in pulse rate. Patients taking high doses or with a history of cardiovascular disease should have ECG monitored before and periodically during therapy.
- **Geri:** Geriatric patients started on trimipramine may be at an increased risk for falls; start with low dose and monitor closely.
- **Depression:** Monitor mental status and affect. Assess for suicidal tendencies, especially during early therapy. Restrict amount of drug available to patient. Risk may be increased in children, adolescents, and adults ≤24 yrs. After starting therapy, children, adolescents, and young adults should be seen by health care professional at least weekly for 4 wks, every 3 wks for next 4 wks, and on advice of health care professional thereafter. Assess for bipolar disorder; onset may

mimic depression and trimipramine is not approved for treatment of bipolar disorder.

- **_Lab Test Considerations:_** Assess leukocyte and differential blood counts, liver function, and serum glucose before and periodically during therapy. May cause an elevated ↑ serum bilirubin and alkaline phosphatase. May cause bone marrow depression. Serum glucose may be increased ↑ or decreased ↓ .

Potential Nursing Diagnoses
Ineffective coping (Indications)
Risk for injury (Side Effects)

Implementation
- Dose increases should be made at bedtime because of sedation. Dose titration is a slow process; may take wk to months. May give entire dose at bedtime. Sedative effect may be apparent before antidepressant effect is noted.
- **PO:** Administer without regards to food.

Patient/Family Teaching
- Instruct patient to take medication as directed. Take missed doses as soon as possible unless almost time for next dose. Advise patient that drug effects may not be noticed for at least 2 wk. Do not discontinue without consulting health care professional. Abrupt discontinuation may cause nausea, vomiting, diarrhea, headache, trouble sleeping with vivid dreams, and irritability. Instruct patient to read medication guide, _Antidepressant Medicines, Depression and other Serious Mental Illness, and Suicidal Thoughts or Actions_ prior to starting therapy and with each Rx refill.

- May cause drowsiness and blurred vision. Caution patient to avoid driving and other activities requiring alertness until response to drug is known.
- Orthostatic hypotension, and sedation are common during early therapy, especially in geriatric patients. Protect patient from falls and advise patient to make position changes slowly.
- Advise patient to avoid alcohol or other CNS depressant drugs during and for 3–7 days after therapy has been discontinued.
- Advise patient and/or family to notify health care professional if anxiety, agitation, panic attacks, insomnia, irritability, hostility, aggressiveness, impulsivity, akathisia, (psychomotor restlessness), hypomania, mania, other unusual changes in behavior, worsening of depression, and suicidal ideation, especially early during antidepressant treatment and when the dose is adjusted up or down.
- Instruct patient to notify health care professional if urinary retention occurs or if dry mouth or constipation persists. Sugarless candy or gum may diminish dry mouth, and an increase in fluid intake or bulk may prevent constipation. If symptoms persist, dose reduction or discontinuation may be necessary. Consult health care professional if dry mouth persists for more than 2 wk.
- Caution patient to use sunscreen and protective clothing to prevent photosensitivity reactions.
- Inform patient of need to monitor dietary intake. Increase in appetite may lead to undesired weight gain.

- Advise patient to notify health care professional if pregnancy is planned or suspected or if breastfeeding.
- Advise patient to notify health care professional of medication regimen before treatment or surgery. Medication should be discontinued as long as possible before surgery.
- Therapy for depression is usually prolonged and should be continued for at least 3 mo to prevent relapse.

Emphasize the importance of follow-up exams to monitor effectiveness and side effects.

Evaluation/Desired Outcomes
- Increased sense of well-being.
- Renewed interest in surroundings.
- Increased appetite.
- Improved energy level.
- Improved sleep.
- Full therapeutic effects may be seen 2–4 wk after initiating therapy.

Table 1 Drugs with New Warnings

Generic name (Brand name)	Warning
Abacavir (Ziagen)	Risk of hypersensitivity reactions in patients with the HLA-B*5701 genetic allele.
Antiepileptic drugs	Risk of suicidality.
Antipsychotics, conventional and atypical	Risk of mortality in elderly patients treated for dementia-related psychoses.
Aprotinin (Trasylol)	Increased mortality; marketing suspended.
Becaplermin (Regranex)	Risk of cancer death.
Clopidogrel (Plavix)	Concurrent use with proton-pump inhibitors may affect drug action.
Darunavir (Prezista)	Risk of hepatotoxicity with ritonavir.
Desmopressin (DDAVP, Minirin, Stimate)	Risk of hyponatremia and seizures.
Efalizumab (Raptiva)	Risk of progressive multifocal leukoencephalopathy (PML).
Epoetin (Epogen, Procrit)	Risk of mortality/tumor progression for some forms of cancer.
Darbepoetin (Aranesp)	Risk of serious cardiovascular/thromboembolic events.
Erlotinib (Tarceva)	Risk of hepatic failure and hepatorenal syndrome, especially in patients with underlying hepatic disease.
Etanercept (Enbrel)	Risk of serious bacterial infections, including sepsis and tuberculosis.

Table 1 (Continued)

Fluoroquinolones	Strengthened warning regarding risk of tendonitis and tendon rupture.
Metoclopramide (Reglan)	Risk of tardive dyskinesia associated with long-term or high dose use.
Over-the-counter cough and cold medications	No longer labeled for use in children under 4 yr of age.
Phenytoin (Dilantin, Phenytek), Fosphenytoin (Cerebyx)	Risk of serious skin reactions including Stevens Johnson syndrome (SJS) and toxic epidermal necrolysis (TEN) from phenytoin therapy in Asian patients positive for HLA-B* 1502. genetic allele.
Efalizumab (Raptiva)	Risk of serious infections including sepsis, meningitis, systemic fungal disease and other potentially fatal infections.
Sodium Phosphate (Visicol, Osmoprep)	Risk of acute phosphate nephropathy.
SSRIs and NSRIs	Risk of neuroleptic malignant syndrome.
Tinzaparin (Innohep)	Mortality risk in elderly patients with renal insufficiency.
Topical anesthetics	Risk of serious adverse reactions (irregular heartbeat, seizures, breathing difficulties, coma and death) when overused.
Transdermal drug patches with metallic backings	Risk of burns to the skin if the patch is worn during an MRI scan.
Tumor necrosis factor-alpha blockers (TNF blockers), Certolizumab (Cimzia), Enbrel (etanercept), Adalimumab (Humira), Infliximab (Remicade)	Risk of disseminated fungal infections.
Varenicline (Chantrix)	Risk of serious neuropsychiatric symptoms including suicidality.
Zanamivir (Relenza), Oseltamivir (Tamiflu)	Risk of delirium and abnormal behavior in children.
Zonisamide (Zonegran)	Risk of metabolic acidosis, especially in younger patients.

Table 2 Drugs with New Dosage Forms or Strengths

Generic name (Brand name)	New dosage form or strength
Amoxicillin (Moxatag)	775 mg extended-release tablet
Bupropion hydrobromide (Aplenzin)	174, 384, and 522 mg extended-release tablets
Calcitriol (Vectical)	3 mcg/g ointment
Ciclesonide (Alvesco)	80 and 160 mcg/inhalation
Fenofibric acid (Trilipix)	45, 135 mg delayed-release oral capsule
Lubiprostone (Amitizia)	8 mcg capsule
Mesalamine (Apriso)	375 mg extended-release capsule
Olopatadine nasal (Patanase)	0.665 mg/spray
Omeprazole (Prilosec)	2.5 and 10 mg/packet for oral suspension
Palonosetron (Aloxi)	0.5 mg capsule
Prednisolone (Flo-Pred)	15 mg/5 mL oral suspension
Prednisolone (Veripred 20)	20 mg/5 mL oral liquid
Risedronate (Actonel)	150 mg tablet
Ropinerole (Requip XL)	2, 3, 4, 8, 12 mg extended-release tablets

Table 2 (Continued)

Generic name (Brand name)	Indication
Temozolomide (Temodar)	100 mg injection
Tretinoin (AtralinGel)	0.05% aqueous gel
Valproic acid (Stavzor)	125, 250, 500 mg delayed-release capsule
Zolpidem (Zolpimist)	5 mg/oral spray

Table 3 Drugs with New Indications

Generic name (Brand name)	New indication
Adalimumab (Humira)	Treatment of moderately- to severely-active polyarticular juvenile idiopathic arthritis in patients ≥4 yr.
Aripiprazole (Abilify)	Acute treatment of manic and mixed episodes associated with Bipolar I Disorder in pediatric patients 10–17 yr old.
Benzyl alcohol lotion, 5%	Treatment of head lice in patients ≥6 mo.
Bevacizumab (Avastin)	Treatment of breast cancer in combination with paclitaxel for patients who have not received chemotherapy for metastatic HER2-negative disease.
Bimatoprost (Latisse)	Promotion of Eyelash growth.
Duloxetine (Cymbalta)	Management of fibromyalgia.
Escitalopram (Lexapro)	Acute/maintenance treatment of major depressive disorder in adolescents 12–17 yr old.
Esomeprazole (Nexium)	Short-term treatment of gastroesophageal reflux disease (GERD) in children ages 1–11 yr.
Fluoxetine (Prozac)	In combination with olanzapine (Zyprexa) for the acute treatment of bipolar depression and treatment-resistant depression (TRD).
Fluoxetine/Olanzapine (Symbyax)	Acute treatment of treatment-resistant depression (TRD).
Fluvoxamine (Luvox CR)	Treatment of social anxiety disorder and obsessive compulsive disorder.
Olanzapine (Zyprexa)	In combination with fluoxetine (Prozac) for the acute treatment of bipolar depression and treatment-resistant depression (TRD).
Tigecycline (Tygacil)	Treatment of community-acquired bacterial pneumonia in adults.

Table 4 New Drug Combinations

Brand name	Components, dosages, and indications
Epiduo	Adapalene 0.1%/benzoyl peroxide 2.5% Management of acne
Kinrix	Diphtheria and tetanus toxoids/acellular pertussis absorbed/inactivated polio vaccine per 0.5 ml dose. Used for the fifth DTaP and fourth dose IPV in 4 to 6 yr olds whose previous DTaP vaccine doses have been with INFANRIX and/or PEDIARIX.
LoSeasonique	84 tablets of 0.1 mg levonorgestrel/0.02 mg ethinyl estradiol and 7 tablets of 0.01 mg ethinyl estradiol Hormonal contraceptive
Prandimet	500 mg metformin/1 mg repaglinide 500 mg metformin/2 mg repaglinide Management of diabetes
Treximet	85 mg sumatriptan/500 mg naproxen tablet Migraine headache

Table 5 Other New Developments

Generic name (Brand name)	Change
Japanese encephalitis vaccine (Ixiaro)	A vaccine for the prevention of Japanese encephalitis (JE), which is caused by a mosquito-transmitted virus found mainly in Asia.